Body *Speak!*

Listen to Your Body...
It Knows What it's Talking About

Michele M. Rizzo, CHC

Certified Integrative Nutrition Health Coach (IIN)

Author, Speaker, Health Educator

For information, email: Michele@michelemrizzo.com

Website: www.michelemrizzo.com

Library of Congress Control Number

ISBN-13: 978-1976348945

ISBN-10: 1976348943

TABLE OF CONTENTS

Dedication   x

Acknowledgements   xi

Medical Disclaimer   xii

A Note from Coach Michele   xiii

PART ONE – *WHAT* Is Happening To Everyone

Chapter 1

This Can't Be Happening!   **3**

A Shocking Wake Up Call   3

The Frightening Cancer Diagnosis   7

Chapter 2

The "C" Word – Facing Fear – Decision Time for The Road Ahead   **9**

Developing a Battle Plan   10

21st Century Healthcare Choices   10

Allopathic Medicine vs. Naturopathic, Holistic and Functional Medicine   11

Chapter 3

Research & Recovery   **17**

The Truth is Out there When You are Determined to find it   18

Dr. Jan's Healing Instructions   18

PART TWO – *WHY*
It's Happening to Everyone

Chapter 4

WHY We All Need to Change the Way We Eat   **23**

SAD – The Standard American Diet is Causing a Health Crisis   24

Food Politics   25

$$$ Government Subsidies   27

Food Value Dollars vs. Health & Quality of Food Choices   28

We Don't Want a Nanny State!   30

Chapter 5

The Misinformation Wars!   **33**

Traversing the WWW.Highway of Misinformation   34

Food Fight! Duck & Cover!   36

Let's Take Soy For Instance   37

Chapter 6

The World is a Dangerous Place – Pesticides, Environment Toxins, GMO's, Factory Farming   **41**

The Dangers of Pesticides   42

Industrial Chemical Invasion – *Bio-sludge!*   43

Cancer is Not Inevitable   45

Misunderstood Connection Between Genes & Cancer   45

Epigenetics and Cancer   47

Genetically Modified Organisms (GMO's)   48

Monsanto GMO Bt-Corn *Itself* is a pesticide!   51

GMO's & Roundup-Ready – Glyphosate   53

Glyphosate & Gluten   55

Leaky Gut Syndrome   55

Celiac Disease   56

Metabolic Belly Fat   57

Cholesterol is Not Your Enemy   58

Top GMO Foods to Avoid – What You Must Eat Organic   59

Organic vs. Conventional Produce   60

Dirty Dozen & Clean Fifteen   60

Factory Farming, Animal Food   61

Antibiotics and Hormones   62

Multi-Drug Resistant Super-Bug Bacteria   64

Chapter 7

Sugar – The Sweet Silent Killer   **65**

Sugar Spikes & Insulin Resistance   67

Sugar is a Highly Addictive Substance   70

Sugar Feeds Cancer   70

Chapter 8

Inflammation – The Fire Within!   **73**

The Immune System   74

Immunization vs. Vaccination   75

The Inflammatory Response   76

Chronic Inflammation – the Link to All Disease   77

PART THREE – *HOW*
To Recover from SAD – Detox & *Thrive!*

Chapter 9

The Anti-Inflammatory Lifestyle   **83**

Acid & Alkaline Forming Foods   83

Grains, Seeds, Nuts   85

Juicing vs. Blending   86

Health Blast Juice Recipe   86

Anti-Inflammatory Supplements & Diet   87

Foods Rich in Antioxidants   88

Chapter 10

The Basics of the Modern Healthy Diet   **89**

A Calorie is a Calorie – Or Is It?   90

Optimal Health & Longevity – The Blue Zones   92

The Mediterranean Diet   94

The Grandmother Effect   95

Chapter 11

The Protein Controversy   **97**

How Much do We Need & What is the Best Source?   97

Marketing Dollars Influence Trends in Nutrition   98

Protein 'Content' How Much do We Need?   99

High Protein – Ketonic Diets   101

Animal Food Proteins   102

Healthy High Protein Choices   102

Vegan Sources of Protein   103

Protein Source Content Chart   106

Chapter 12

Probiotics & Fermented Foods that Heal   107

Probiotics   108

Seven Reasons to Eat Fermented Foods   109

Top Ten Fermented Foods   109

Chapter 13

Detox & Colon Health   111

What is Detox?   112

Why Detox?   113

A Clean Colon is a Healthy Colon   114

Clinical Constipation – *SERIOUS Danger*
of Developing Colon Cancer   116

Constipation is Dehydration   116

Electromagnetic Radiation – EMR   118

Chapter 14

How to DETOX   **121**

Detoxing from Chemotherapy, Drugs & Radiation   122

Detox Do's and Do Not's   123

Detoxing Body Systems   125

Skin Detox Epson Salt Recipe   129

Drink Lemon Water Routine for Daily Natural Detox Benefits   131

Detoxing the Colon   132

Vegetable Juice Combinations   133

Heavy Metal Removal Smoothie Recipes   133

Detox Recipe Combinations   135

Choosing a Juice Only Fast   137

Breaking a Juice Only Fast   139

Chapter 15 – Getting Started on A New Road to Health!

The Elimination Detox & Diet   **141**

Gentle Detox – What to Expect   143

3 Meals a Day – No Snacks   144

Blood Sugar Balancing   145

The Crowding Out Method   147

Emotional Check-In & Self Inquiry   148

After 21-Day EDD   150

Food Allergies vs. Food Sensitivities   150

Chapter 16

EDD Acceptable Foods Shopping & Cooking Guides

EDD Acceptable Foods Shopping & Cooking Guides — 151

Plant-based Vegan Tastes vs. SAD Animal Food Tastes — 152

Elimination Detox Diet Food Guide — 153

Healthy Cooking Guidelines — 158

Soaking & Cooking Grains — 161

Soaking & Sprouting Beans — 162

Culinary Spices from Around the World — 164

Basic Vegan Shopping List — 166

Kitchen Tools — 167

Chapter 17

Standard American Diet Recovery Bootcamp

Standard American Diet Recovery Bootcamp — 169

Successfully Navigating the Busy Work Week — 169

Create an EDD Seven-Day Meal Plan — 172

7-Day EDD Sample Meal Plan — 174

Chapter 18

Elimination Detox & Diet Recipes

Elimination Detox & Diet Recipes — 179

EDD Breakfast Inspirations — 181

EDD Salad Entrée's Selections — 192

Savory EDD Soup Entrée Selections — 205

EDD Main Meal Entrée Selections — 213

AFTER EDD Food Re-Introduction 236

Slowly Re-Introduce Eliminated Foods 236

Where to Go Now 237

Chapter 19

AFTER EDD Delicious Healthy Recipes **239**

A Few Favorite Go-To Recipes 240

On The Sweet Side 255

Chapter 20

Reliable Health Resources **267**

Michele M. Rizzo Health Coaching Services 268

Cancer 270

Detox & Healing Chronic Illness 271

Educational Health & Nutrition 272

Reliable Laboratories for Nutraceuticals & Supplements 272

RECIPE INDEX

EDD Breakfast Selections 273

EDD Lunch Entrée Selections 274

EDD Savory Soup Entrée Selections 275

EDD Main Meal Selections 275

AFTER EDD – Delicious Healthy Recipes 277

A Few 'Go-To' Favorites 277

On The Sweet Side 278

Dedication

With overflowing gratitude I dedicate this book to all the courageous true healers of the world. The unsung heroes of health who pave the way for the rest of us to follow.

To those who pay a price for speaking the truth in a world of ridicule, contempt, misinformation and downright lies.

Together we can take our health back, rescue the planet and make a difference.

ACKNOWLEDGMENTS

We thank Dr. Jan for taking the time to help us in our hour of desperate need. Thank you for leading the way to help us find the true healers in this world – and for being one yourself!

We acknowledge all of our loving, praying, caring family and friends who stood with us every step of the way. Janet, for your generous gift of the Kangen water system and nightly calls of love and encouragement. Your solid support of me as a Health Coach and book author. Thank you. Deb & Dave for racing to our side to be with us during the surgical procedure and standing with us through thick and thin!

Lynn, thank you for your loving support and opening your home to me when Mike was in the hospital. Your tangible strength and love carried us through this difficult season.

Linda, Tony & Doreen thank you for coming up to Arrowhead and praying for Mike when he was so sick. That prayer time was a turning point in Mike's recovery.

Thank you Zach for grocery shopping for all those challenging organic ingredients and bringing them up to us when Dad was too sick to be alone and I couldn't leave him to grocery shop.

To our wonderful children Ben, Zach and Allison who love us unconditionally and stand with us in support of all the difficult and inspiring lifestyle changes.

Thank you Sandee and Mom for reading this book and offering your editorial input and proofreading skill.

I acknowledge my beloved Michael's courageous choice to fight this life-threatening illness by embracing nutrition and making a total lifestyle overhaul rather than giving up in despair and allowing disease to take your life prematurely.

I acknowledge all the amazing, creative and inspirational plant-based cooks and bloggers who share their recipes with the world. I never would have figured out the wonders of cashew cream, nutritional yeast, flaxseed 'eggs' and chickpea flour!

I acknowledge the Institute of Integrative Nutrition (IIN) for the excellent and professional training I received to become a Certified Nutritional Health Coach.

Medical Disclaimer

THE ELIMINATION DETOX DIET PROGRAM

Isolating Food Sensitivities, Allergies & Correcting Digestive Disorders

The *Elimination Detox Diet (EDD)* is a unique program written by Integrative Nutrition Health Coach, Michele M. Rizzo. Michele trained with leading health professionals of our day through the Institute of Integrative Nutrition (IIN). She is certified through the American Academy of Drugless Practitioners.

The EDD does not include any supplementation, powders or pills. It simply eliminates some of the foods that are difficult to digest in order to identify whether or not these foods are the cause of digestive issues.

This program has been designed to help you reset your body clock, naturalize your weight and gently detox your body. This program is not designed to diagnose or heal serious illness such as diabetes, heart disease or cancer.

All material provided in the *Elimination Detox Diet* program is for informational or educational purposes only. Schedule a consultation with your naturopathic practitioner, or your doctor for specific medical diagnoses and recommendations to treat illness.

Continue taking all prescribed medications while following the *EDD* program.

When you eliminate hard to digest food, and begin to eat clean, organic fruits and vegetables, your body will naturally detox and release weight. You may experience some detox symptoms – which are described a little later on – but these symptoms will go away within a few days and you will experience more energy and vitality while eating and following this diet protocol.

If you are on diuretics or diabetes medication, have liver or gallbladder disease, or have any serious health concerns, please proceed only under doctor's supervision.

A Note From Coach Michele

Congratulations! You are embarking on a life-changing journey toward health, vitality, and wellbeing! Good for you. I am so happy you are here and joining me on this odyssey of health and discovery.

'Body Speak!' is learning how to listen to your body and understand what it is telling you. Symptoms are signals your body is sending to help you understand what it needs to be healthy and strong. Symptoms are the body's only way of communication, so it is vital to learn how to listen and respond to these cries for help.

Body speak signals are symptoms that present in varying levels of severity from headache, fever and heartburn to obesity, diabetes, kidney failure, heart disease and cancer.

Our bodies are amazing bio-machines created to optimize health and vitality. When given the right ingredients and proper care, our bodies have the opportunity to heal, thrive and live long healthy lives.

In 2015, my husband Mike was diagnosed with cholangiocarcinoma, a rare and deadly cancer with scant medical options for recovery. Our world changed forever that day. Surprisingly, for the better. Our journey from deadly cancer diagnosis to the clean bill of health Mike enjoys today is the subject of this book. This is the book I wish I had then, when we felt like we were tossed off a cliff into a dark pit.

When Mike became ill, we turned to our friend, Dr. Jan, a naturopathic doctor. At that time, we were 'health-illiterate', scared, and needing all the help we could get!

Dr. Jan set us on a course toward health through nutrition and lifestyle changes. We did everything she told us to, and more. She encouraged us to learn from the leading natural health practitioners of our time. She sent us links to articles, videos and books that would teach and train us how to recover our health and vitality. We learned to 'tune in' to what our bodies were telling us.

Dr. Jan told Mike to cut out all sugar and meat to enable his body to recover from its health crisis. She suggested a raw diet so we decided to go vegan together. A vegan diet is void of all animal products, including dairy and eggs. Nothing that comes from any living being, other than a plant. We never considered going vegan before, but we are so glad we did. The health benefits we both enjoy after making our lifestyle changes are surprising and amazing.

Before Mike's diagnosis, he was taking Statins for high cholesterol, blood pressure medication, and Prilosec for his constant heartburn. His body was desperately crying out for help. We did not know how to read the signs of imminent failure until it was almost too late. By treating symptoms with pharmaceuticals rather than addressing the underlying root causes, Mike's body was heading down the inevitable path toward early death.

I made Mike's cancer diagnosis an opportunity for my own health intervention as well. My body was sending me signals that my lifestyle was leading me toward degenerative decline. I suffered from high blood pressure, insomnia, heartburn and carried extra weight. I was also masking these 'body speak' symptoms with pharmaceuticals.

After a few months of enjoying this new lifestyle, I lost weight, my blood pressure was back to normal, and I felt great. I know I will never gain weight back because I've learned how to make delicious and nutritious whole food meals that are filling, satisfying and naturally weight balancing.

Today, we are healthier, stronger, and experiencing more vitality than we have in years due to implementing the changes I share with you in this book. We did it all naturally and no longer need to take any pharmaceuticals. Mike and I have not remained strictly vegan. We eat organic and enjoy occasional wild-caught seafood.

Mike's recovery through diet and nutrition is a testimony to the healing power of food as medicine. Also, we thank God daily for Mike's healing. We relied heavily on the healing power of God's amazing grace during this battle.

Research reveals, that cancer is linked to both genetic and environmental factors. It is said, *"Genes load the gun, but the environment pulls the trigger."* Mike's cancer diagnosis was most likely linked to eating today's unhealthy, toxic, pesticide and chemical ridden foods. We always thought we ate healthy – mostly home cooked meals, lots of chicken, and low-carb paleo meals. Not too much processed, fried or junk food. Mike didn't eat in-between meals and maintained a healthy body weight. He went to the gym regularly and led an active life. The cancer diagnosis shocked us. Why did Mike get cancer? We will discuss this in depth later.

If you or a loved one are fighting cancer or other major disease right now, I do not claim to have a *cure* for you. However, when we give our bodies everything they need to heal, and remove the toxins in our body and environment, we have a fighting chance to recover. Choosing to eat an organic, mostly plant based diet is choosing to live a cancer-preventative lifestyle.

This is not a *"how to survive cancer"* book, but rather how to treat our body with the best love, care and nutrition available to prevent cancer, chronic disease, and the degenerative ailments that come with age.

When we live an informed, proactive lifestyle of health and nutrition, it is possible to age with grace, dignity and full mental capacity. There is no need to degenerate into fragile breaking bones, loss of mobility, incontinence and senility. Age alone does not cause these consequences, but living a sedentary lifestyle and eating the Standard American Diet (SAD) loaded with toxic pesticides, high fructose corn syrup, factory farmed meat, sugar, GMO's and chemicals, does.

If you are fighting cancer and have already gone through the traditional methods of treatment with chemotherapy and radiation, you need to recover from the damages these treatments have done to your body. It is suggested you remove all toxic food from your diet and detox your body – gently – as described here. Nourish and strengthen your immune system with fresh organic juices and lots of raw fruits and vegetables. Heal your gut by eating organic fermented foods. When you do this, you give your body a fighting chance to heal and recover health.

Through research and deciphering my own 'Body Speak' signals, I now relate to food in a new light. I no longer look at food as the number of calories I consume, but rather, the amount of toxins and sugar I am putting into my body. Now that I understand what my body must go through when I mistreat it with harmful food, I no longer *choose* to do so. I am free, empowered and happy to make food decisions that will not only nourish me, but slow down the aging process and fend off serious illness and loss of mobility in my later years.

These days, when I am at a potluck function or restaurant I am conscious of what I am putting into my body and how much harm I may be doing to myself. In the past, when I gave myself 'permission' to indulge, it would be whatever was on that potluck table, or whatever I wanted to order off a menu. Now that I tune in to my own 'Body Speak,' and act accordingly, I am enjoying a new, profound appreciation for my body and health. I am choosing to love myself with the food I eat. This is a new and liberating way to live and I am loving it.

The best way to learn 'Body Speak,' is to go on the **Elimination Detox Diet (EDD)**, chapters 15-18 of this book. This program detoxifies your body naturally and locates specific foods that may be causing distress. The EDD trains you to listen to the signals your body is sending and how to respond with healing nutrition and protocols.

The EDD is not 'easy' – but it is doable! If you need some extra support – give me a shout out – I'll help you. I've added delicious and satisfying recipes in this book that will go a long way in helping you achieve your health goals. There are multiple health benefits for going on the EDD. It has the power to unlock mysteries and get to the root cause of digestive issues, food sensitivities and allergic reactions that you may suffer from unaware.

REMEMBER – I am here for you! I love to connect and answer questions. You can check out my health coach practice by going to my website: www.michelemrizzo.com. I conduct periodic online health courses and group coaching circles. Go online to check out the schedule of upcoming events. You can also subscribe to receive my informative and inspiring newsletters. I offer complimentary Health Histories, personal Skype or Facetime sessions, and 6-month, personally guided health programs. Contact me today and together, we'll work up some health goals that will get you on your way to a lifetime of health, and vitality.

As the wise saying goes - *Health is a Journey – Not a Destination.* **You can't lose – if you don't quit!**

To your health & success!

Coach Michele

- Part One -
WHAT
Is Happening to Everyone?

Chapter 1

This Can't Be Happening!

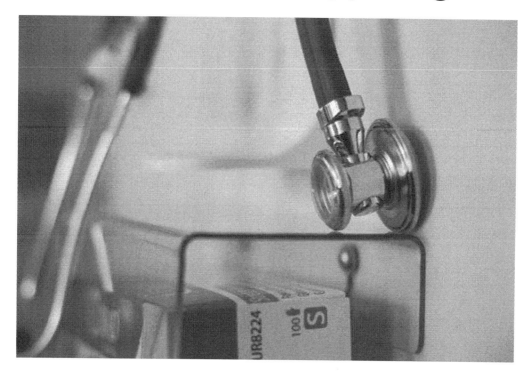

A Shocking Wake Up Call

We entered the hospital emergency room before dawn. A janitor bobbed his head to the beat coming from his headphones as he moved a whirling floor buffer around in circles. Parents fussed with a crying toddler, while another mother gently rocked her sleeping child. A coughing, sneezing woman, wrapped in a blanket sat huddled in a chair. I wrapped my own scarf around my nose and mouth in a vain attempt to ward off the germs.

After turning in the paperwork we took our seats. I took out my phone to text the family who were all on high alert for news regarding Mike's emergency gallbladder surgery. I updated them we were checked in and waiting to see the doctor. I assured everyone I would notify them as soon as Mike went in for surgery.

Mike took my hand and held tight. We leaned our heads close and discussed softly the alarming events of the past few weeks.

Life had finally calmed down. Our three wonderful kids were grown with busy lives of their own. We were finding one another again, having fun and enjoying our new home in Lake Arrowhead. Our life had reverted to what it was like as newlyweds, but with the maturity and wisdom that only the years can bring.

Mike was learning to cook more than grilling meat on the BBQ. We loved turning on our favorite music and dancing around the kitchen while cooking together. We enjoyed nice wine and talked for hours into the night. We were falling in love afresh, discovering the depth of one another in ways that we were unable to do before while raising kids and building careers. This little gallbladder surgery was a mere hiccup on the path to a bright, long future together.

"Mike Rizzo," the nurse called, it was time to go in.

The emergency room doctor began asking questions and Mike talked him through his recent health history. How over the past couple months his appetite dwindled and his feet and entire body began to itch incessantly. When he started to turn yellow, the alarm bells went off. So he went into his primary physician for X-rays and blood work.

"What did the tests say?" asked the doctor.

"Well, the ultrasound suggested either a liver tumor or an enlarged gallbladder. My doctor suggested I have my gallbladder out," Mike answered.

This had been a week earlier, and by the time Mike presented in the emergency room he was *extremely* yellow. The whites of his eyes were close to the color of mustard. His skin had broken out into sores all over his legs, arms and torso. He was miserable.

"Do you have any pain in your abdomen?"

"No," Mike replied.

"What color are your stools?"

"Chalky white," Mike answered.

"How much weight have you lost?"

"I've lost 65 pounds."

"In how much time?" the doctor asked as he looked up from his paperwork.

Mike looked at me, and then back to the doctor. "I would have to say about three weeks."

The doctor took off his reading glasses and looked Mike straight in his eyes. "When a man of your age presents in the emergency room, yellow, with skin lesions, white stools, dropping so much weight in such a short period of time and no abdominal pain, it is not your gallbladder. Let me assure you, if it was your gallbladder you would be screaming in pain, vomiting and demanding surgery."

Taking a brief pause he said it straight out, "No. I'm afraid what we are looking at here is pancreatic cancer."

We were stunned.

"I apologize for shocking you like this, but in emergency room medicine, we go from the worst case scenario and work backwards. I'll order all the tests, and we'll go from there." He called in the nurse and gave her the orders. He told her he wanted to talk personally to the ultrasound technician before the ultrasound was given. She agreed and waved us to come along with her.

We followed the nurse into the back working lab area, and she handed Mike a urine sample cup. As he left the room, she got busy on her computer. A few minutes later Mike came around the corner holding his urine sample, and honestly, it was the color of espresso coffee. I gasped. The nurse was visibly taken aback at the color of Mike's urine. It was a bad omen of things to come.

The nurse had Mike sit in a wheelchair and allowed me to accompany them to the ultrasound. We waited there with the technician until the doctor came in and instructed the tech to take extra time and pictures around the biliary tree. They talked in medical jargon we didn't understand. The friendly tech explained to us what the doc wanted and showed us the biliary tree while he conducted the ultrasound. The biliary tree is a system of vessels that direct the digestive secretions from the liver, gallbladder and pancreas through a series of ducts into the duodenum. This series of ducts connect these vital organs and bears some resemblance to a tree – thus the name; biliary tree.

We were like a couple scared kids not understanding a single thing we were looking at, but hoping the tech would say – *"Hey guys, it all looks good to me!"* He didn't.

The MRI and intravenous renal scan were next; both these tests require radiation, so I was led to a small waiting area where a few others sat watching TV. Soon the ER doctor came to find me.

We stood to the side and talked in hushed tones.

"The initial tests have come back in. I am still waiting for the intravenous renal scan results. It may take an hour or two for those. I've put a rush on everything. I'm afraid I need to tell you we are looking at pancreatic cancer."

I stood rigid and crossed my arms – internally asking God for strength. I knew that there are two "p" cancers men get; pancreatic and prostate. Prostate cancer has pretty good odds of recovery, but pancreatic cancer? Not so much.

"If this is the case, how long do you think he has to live?" I asked.

"Well, it is premature for me to say exactly, but I would have to say you are looking at about six months."

There it was; the bomb. I went cold. The room took on a surreal bluish hue. *God will help me*, I thought. *This can't be happening.*

At a loss for words I lamely thanked him for coming to find me and letting me know. He just nodded sadly and walked out. The nurse came in, led me to the patient section of the emergency room, and gave me a chair next to the bed Mike would occupy after the tests. She asked if she could get me anything and I asked for a warm blanket, I felt chilled to the bone.

I took out my cell phone and began texting our prayer brigade. We have a strong network of faith-filled; prayer warrior family and friends and we needed their help, big time. I sent texts to our three children letting them know we were not looking at emergency gallbladder surgery, but a very serious potential cancer diagnosis. I chose not to tell them what the doctor had said, but to warn them it was bad news.

A tech wheeled Mike to his bed and settled him in. We just held each other for a few moments. We hadn't had a chance to talk since the frightening words; "pancreatic cancer" had been spoken.

"You can't go to heaven and leave me alone in this crazy world," I whispered. I chose not tell Mike yet about the six-month death sentence the doctor had pronounced.

He just held me. I put myself in his shoes and felt the fear and shock of it all.

"Now, I know what Paul is feeling," he said. Mike's brother Paul had bladder cancer. Mike called his brother and they both cried together on the phone.

It is one thing to support a loved one dying from cancer; it is a whole other thing to now be faced with a cancer diagnosis too. The brothers put their phones on speaker so the wives could join in the conversation. The four of us loved on each other, and softly wept together. Mike's brother Paul passed from cancer three months later.

The Frightening Diagnosis

When all the test results came in, the ER doctor came back to tell us his diagnosis. It was *cholangiocarcinoma*, a rare and deadly cancer of the bile ducts. It was not the pancreatic cancer he first thought, but something more rare, and deadly. No one recovers from this cancer through traditional treatments. I know because I looked them all up *(later not that day)*. The best you can hope for is some borrowed time through chemotherapy, and in extreme cases a liver transplant.

Mike's body was unable to eliminate the toxins building up in his liver because they could not get past the abnormal cells blocking his bile ducts. His life was threatened by this deadly toxin build-up. This is why his skin broke out in sores. It was his body's desperate attempt to get rid of toxins in order to save his life. Without the expertise and intervention of modern medicine, Mike would soon go into kidney failure and die.

The doctor wanted Mike to have an Endoscopic Retrograde Cholangio-Pancreatography, (ERCP), a procedure used to examine diseases of the liver, bile ducts, and pancreas. During this procedure they would take a biopsy and insert a "stent" which would hold the bile duct open to drain out the toxins in the liver. The stent would be eliminated from the body in several weeks.

The doctor began making phone calls to get Mike admitted into Loma Linda University, the leading cancer treatment center in the area. He felt we were dealing with such a delicate procedure he wanted a highly experienced "tumor team" to perform the ERCP. I heard him calling in favors from his colleagues while pacing in the corridor on his cell phone. Loma Linda is a notoriously over crowded hospital in much demand for its expertise and skill, but the ER doctor was able to get Mike admitted.

We called our two sons and daughter to tell them the shocking news. No, Dad is not getting his gallbladder out today. He is being transported to Loma Linda Medical University for an emergency ERCP because he has deadly cholangiocarcinoma and his bile ducts are completely blocked.

Mike told them NOT to Google cholangiocarcinoma. Our sons did not take their dad's advice. They both Googled it, and were devastated. Our daughter told her boss she was no longer able to function and left work, fighting the commute traffic to get to us as soon as she could.

Mike had Googled *cholangiocarcinoma* while we waited for the transport. I didn't let him tell me what it said. I did not want to hear it. It was all too soon and fresh for me. I put my trust in God and knew there had to be a way to beat it. ***I was not about to accept this death sentence lying down.***

The ERCP was performed the following day. Mike spent three nights in the hospital. We are so grateful for the medical expertise and care Mike received at Loma Linda University. Without the ERCP surgical procedure, Mike would not have survived. We could feel God's peace and grace with us every step of the way.

But damn, we were scared.

Chapter 2

The "C" Word - Facing Fear and Decision Time for the Road Ahead

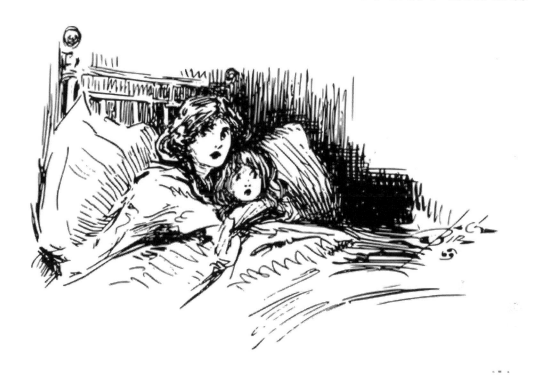

Cancer, the dreaded "C" word — I don't know of another word that strikes more terror in the heart than hearing a doctor say, "*It's cancer.*"

Cancer is rising in alarming rates. It is estimated now — world wide — that one in three people will get a cancer diagnosis in their lifetime. These are staggering odds. You or someone you love might be fighting this or another deadly disease right now and this is why you are reading this book. There is hope, I promise. This book is loaded with helpful information to get you started on the road to recovery. Never give up. Use this book as a resource, and check out all the other books and links I share in the Appendix to help you. You are not alone. Many people have walked this road and are alive today to tell their story of victory. You can too.

Developing A Battle Plan

We started investigating our options to begin fighting for Mike's life. This led us onto a path of discovery and understanding that cancer and many other deadly diseases afflicting our modern society are mainly caused by our toxic environment and lifestyle choices. Not just bad luck or genetics. To overcome these diseases we need to find the source of the problem, remove it, and allow our bodies to eradicate the disease and heal. This journey is not for the faint of heart, but it works.

> **Our bodies are not *drug deficient*, they are stressed from poisons in our food and water and suffering from malnutrition – even as we are quickly becoming the most obese society in history.**

21ST CENTURY HEALTHCARE CHOICES AVAILABLE

In today's world of modern medicine there are two approaches to disease:

1) The "Germ Theory of Disease," authored by Louis Pasteur, and

2) The "Cellular Theory of Disease," authored by Antoine Bechamp.

The Germ Theory of Disease: believes that germs, including viruses and bacteria, are bad and that they are the cause of all disease and illness. This is the foundation of Western (*Allopathic*) Medicine.

Based on this assumption, killing germs is the solution for preventing and treating *all* disease. The germ theory is the foundation of the entire pharmaceutical industry's legal drug cartel. The industry has morphed from killing germs – to creating drugs to squelch 'Body Speak' signals by attacking every symptom the body manifests with synthetic chemicals.

The Cellular Theory of Disease: believes infection from germs is a 'result' of a compromised immune system, not the 'cause' of the illness. When the body becomes damaged due to high toxic load and poor lifestyle choices, opportunistic germs overcome the broken down immune system and cause symptoms to manifest and disease to take root.

The Cellular Theory of Disease does not advocate the killing of germs – but rather the cultivation of health and strengthening the immune system through detoxification, nutrition, hygiene and healthy lifestyle practices. Germs will not sicken a person if they are in good health. This is the foundation of naturopathic, holistic and functional medicine.

Allopathic Medicine vs. Naturopathic, Holistic and Functional Medicine

Allopathic – Western Medicine

Medical doctors are trained to specialize in one part of the body and combat disease by the use of drugs or surgery. Allopathic medicine does not treat the whole person with natural means, nor does it seek the root cause of disease for a cure. The human body is dissected into various medical 'specialties' i.e. cardiology, neurology, pulmonology, psychology, OBGYN, orthopedics, etc. depending on the symptoms. These specialists all use different drug applications to suppress symptoms.

Who Needs a Cure? Pills are Big Business!

This philosophy ascribes to the belief humans are the product of their genes and victim to germs; therefore there is no need to look for the root source of disease or modify our lifestyle choices. Just sterilize everything, get your annual flu shot, keep the kids up to date with their vaccines and take doctor prescribed pharmaceuticals to knock down discomfort and distressing symptoms (*forget those annoying body speak signals*). Who wants to suffer, just give us a pill, right?

"One pill makes you larger, and one pill makes you small, and the ones that mother gives you, don't do anything at all. Go ask Alice, when she's ten feet tall"

Jefferson Airplane.

"*Ask your doctor,*" the TV pill pushers say. In the past, advertising drugs directly to consumers was illegal, but big pharma got past that one and now places attractive people in drug commercials lobbying for your business. Especially during the nightly news, a veritable plethora of the latest and greatest drugs are paraded for solicitation. Everything from leaky bladder to penile dysfunction. All you have to do is get your allopathic doctor to prescribe the latest and greatest patented pill. Just take this synthetic chemical concoction and go on enjoying life as usual with no "sane" intervention for lasting health.

"Whack-A-Mole" The Game of 'Patented' Symptom Suppressors

Allopathic medicine can be compared to the arcade game – *"Whack-A-Mole."* A doctor prescribes one medicine, thus hitting the presenting symptom, the 'mole' on the head with a hammer, only to have another 'mole' or 'symptom' pop up in its place. One drug after another is used in an endless attempt to squelch symptoms. Your body is sending you these body speak symptoms in an attempt to get you to address the underlying cause. By suppressing the symptoms, the root cause is not addressed and will worsen, becoming diabetes, heart disease, kidney failure and cancer.

> # The problem with pharmaceutical drugs is – they are chemicals that have serious side effects and actually cause disease and even cancer.

Pills might help with initial symptoms, but they don't cure disease at the root cause. Pharmaceutical drugs come with a vast array of side-effects. Some of them worse than the original presenting condition. Begin to notice the marketing manipulation of TV drug commercials. The appealing actors are all smiling, and so relieved to be on this 'wonderful' drug. As the commercial ends, the volume of the announcer's voice is purposely turned low and then it speeds up to the point of near incoherence while listing a wide range of possible alarming side effects – all the way from headaches, to blindness and in some cases *death*!

Eat This Pill Rainbow America!

Go ahead over weight sick America, eat that chili dog, nachos and fries just be sure to take that little purple pill every day so you won't be bothered with annoying heartburn and indigestion. Block that 'evil' stomach acid causing you distress, after all, who needs stomach acid to digest their food? We've got you covered. Heaven forbid you learn how to eat and NOT get heartburn.

And for you men out there not able to get erect for sex? We've got you covered! Just take the little blue pill, and if you get an erection lasting longer than four hours call your doctor. Oh and did we forget to tell you? Often erectile dysfunction is a sign of an underlying vascular condition that could be affecting your heart.

Erectile Dysfunction could be a sign you are approaching a heart attack, or stroke, or diabetes. But don't worry about all that – our little 'blue' pill has you covered!   Even your GP can prescribe it!

Modern western medicine has saved millions of lives. When we are in a car accident, or need broken bones fixed, or require emergency life-saving surgical interventions, these are the experts trained to help us. And we need them.

Antibiotics and pharmaceutical interventions are necessary and life-saving in the right circumstances. However, being on pills for long periods of time to treat chronic illness can lead to other serious issues and degenerative disorders.

Sadly, it is reported today by a multiple of sources that the third leading cause of death in the United States – after cancer and heart disease - is caused by medical error. Unwarranted surgeries, drug complications, misdiagnosis and superbug anti-biotic resistant germs in hospitals.

Allopathic – Oncology; Cancer Treatment

Once cancer is found, the patient is referred to oncology which is the study and treatment of tumors. Traditional oncological methods of treating cancer are surgery, chemotherapy or radiation. In some cases all three are used in the course of treatment.

Unfortunately, at the present time, there are no other options offered in the allopathic approach to treating cancer. Your options are; cut, poison or burn. Which will it be? All three? Coming right up! And the sooner the better, because after all, this horrible disease already has a leg up on you, it's time to attack it! Cancer must be nuked, poisoned or cut out. Period. Nothing else is offered.

If chemotherapy and/or radiation are the treatments you or a loved one have chosen to combat cancer, then it is wise to couple these treatments with good solid detox and nutrition to help build the immune system to withstand chemotherapy and fight the disease.

It is very important to rid the body of toxins after chemotherapy treatments. Seeking the guidance of a Functional Medicine Doctor or Naturopathic Doctor trained in nutrition and detox can help you do this safely and under proper supervision.

> ### *"Functional Medicine is the Medicine of Why."*
> ### *Dr. Mark Harmon.*

Functional Medicine

Functional Medicine is a new breed of medical doctor trained to address the underlying causes of disease. It uses a systems-oriented approach engaging both patient and practitioner in a therapeutic partnership.

Dr. Mark Harmon, Functional Medicine Doctor and top selling author explains:

"Functional Medicine is the future of conventional medicine — available now. It seeks to identify and address the root causes of disease, and views the body as one integrated system, not a collection of independent organs divided up by medical specialties. It treats the whole system, not just the symptoms."

Naturopathic Medicine

Naturopathic medicine is an approach to health care that uses natural, non-toxic therapies to treat the whole person and encourage the self-healing process.

Natural and naturopathic therapies include:

- **Herbal and botanical preparations**, such as herbal extracts and teas
- **Dietary supplements**, such as vitamins, minerals and amino acids
- **Homeopathic remedies**, extremely low doses of plant extracts and minerals
- **Physical therapy and exercise therapy**, including massage and other gentle techniques used on deep muscles and joints for therapeutic purposes
- **Hydrotherapy**, which prescribes water-based approaches like hot and cold wraps, and other therapies
- **Lifestyle counseling**, such as exercise, sleep strategies, stress reduction techniques, as well as foods and nutritional supplements
- **Acupuncture**, to help with side effects like nausea and vomiting, dry mouth, hot flashes and insomnia
- **Chiropractic care**, which may include hands-on adjustment, massage, stretching, electronic muscle stimulation, traction, heat, ice and other techniques

Homeopathy

Homeopathy is a system of medical practice making use of all measures available that prove valuable in the treatment of disease. Nutrition, herbs, meditation, tinctures and massage therapy are among these healing modalities.

A herbalist is a person trained and licensed in treating illness with medicinal herbs. Herbs are used as medicine to treat and heal underlying health issues. Herbs do not work as quickly to mask symptoms in the say way that pharmaceutical drugs do, so people need to be patient and trust in the process of healing. Herbs and proper nutrition heal the body by addressing the underlying cause of illness and disease. Pharmaceutical drugs mask body speak symptoms and do not address the underlying reason of why these symptoms showed up in the first place.

OUR CHOICE – THE ALL NATURAL ROUTE - NO CHEMO OR RADIATION

After Mike was released from the hospital the Loma Linda surgeon called to discuss options. He had written orders for Mike to receive follow-up care in the oncology (cancer) department, but in the meantime he wanted Mike to come in for more tests and another ERCP. The surgeon explained that the ERCP procedure can be done up to three times in order to keep the bile ducts flowing. He cautioned Mike not to wait too long as his condition was aggressive.

Oncology only offers chemotherapy and radiation. These were not options Mike wanted to take because these two approaches are destructive to the body and offer no guarantee for lasting recovery for this type of cancer.

The ERCP worked to open Mike's clogged bile ducts, and the toxins slowly drained out of his body. Thankfully, the itching stopped almost immediately. He looked like a yellow – pink swirled soft-serve ice cream cone as his yellow skin slowly faded and his normal skin tone returned. Mike was still weak and sick, but the ERCP was a life-saving intervention, without it he would not have lasted much longer.

We followed all of the instructions given to us by our naturopathic doctor – as described in Chapter 3. We also prayed together every day and Mike slowly recovered.

Three months after the ERCP Mike returned to his primary physician and the CA-19-9 cancer antigen test for pancreatic cancer came back normal! His doctor was amazed and so happy for him. Mike told him everything he had been doing and he replied, *"It's amazing what you can do with a gun to your head. Keep up the good work and stay healthy."* Mike was able to return to the gym within six months of his illness. It took about a year for him to gain back the weight he had lost. Today, he is doing fantastic and enjoying life to the fullest.

Chapter 3

Research & Recovery

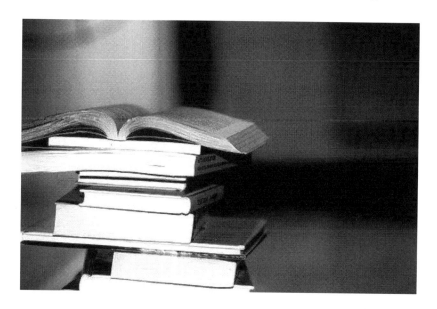

> ***This is the book I wish I had back then. I had NO IDEA of where to start – or what to do.***

From the list of health care options described in Chapter 2, we chose to continue to consult our friend Jan, a Naturopathic Doctor. We did *everything* Dr. Jan told us to do, and more. She sent us links to natural health healers who have been treating people – with amazing results – for years. I searched out all the links she sent me, and discovered more along the way.

My curiosity sent me into researching the *why* behind Dr. Jan's instructions. I searched for doctors who have been 'healing' people for 30 – 40 years; I figured these are the people who know what they are talking about in the area of health and nutrition.

> # The truth is out there when you are determined to find it. Once found – believe the truth and do what it says.

Dr. Jan's Natural Healing Instructions:

- Drink Lou Corona's *'Ginger Blast'* juice two to three times a day; free recipe found online
- Stop eating sugar
- Stop eating meat
- Stop eating processed food
- Eat raw blended 'soups' – no spice
- Eat organic vegan
- DETOX!
- Drink baking soda & molasses & black cumin oil 2 times daily
- Educate yourself!

We started with *'Ginger Blast'* juice but then began adding beets and other ingredients we felt were nutritious and helpful. The juice recipe we came up with we call; *'Health Blast Juice'* because it is not a sweet, tasty juice. It's packed full of nutrition, so when it's ready to drink – we lift our glasses for a toast to life and chuck it down! This recipe can be found on page 184. I also go into more detail of why no sugar and meat later.

We faithfully followed Dr. Jan's instructions and Mike began recovering. In a few short months he was regaining weight and his blood test for the pancreatic cancer antigen came back normal. It was incredible! From being at death's door, and hearing he probably only had six months to live – to today being 100% cancer free is remarkable! It still took Mike over a year to fully recover but now we are both healthier than we've been in years.

Transitioning to an Upgraded Life of Health and Nutrition

When Dr. Jan told us to eat vegan – I had to come up with a whole new way of cooking. I began searching for vegan recipes, reading natural healing articles and watching YouTube video interviews from leading natural health practitioners of our day. There was a ton of information, and I was clueless but hungry to learn both the 'why' and 'how' to live a healthy lifestyle.

The prevailing thought 'out there' among folks who are not health conscious is that vegans are weirdos and health food tastes bloody awful. Who wants to eat like a rabbit and drink slimy greens mixed up in a blender? Boring. Yuck. Life is too short, I'll take my chances, eat what I want, maybe exercise a bit here and there – and hope for the best.

Considering today's toxic food supply, this kind of thinking will get you killed – at a much younger age than necessary.

> *Our life required a TOTAL overhaul in how we ate and related to food and our health. I'll be honest; this is not easy to do. But it IS doable. And having this book filled with the 'why' and 'how' will help you too as you travel this journey toward health and wholeness.*

We had a long way to go and didn't know it

When Mike got sick, we *believed* we were eating pretty well. His life before the cancer diagnosis consisted of a nightly Scotch and a cigar. Meals were mostly home cooked and centered around beef or chicken. Not salmon or fish, Mike never cared for it and cooking fish stunk up the whole house – so when fish was eaten it was out at a fancy restaurant. Dinner was followed up with a bowl of ice cream every night, sometimes served on top of hot baked pie. All that ultra-health and nutrition stuff was for the 'other guy.' There was no need to worry about all that. Mike was going to the gym three times a week and feeling great; rarely ever sick –

until the worst of the worst happened and he was diagnosed with cancer - what a rude awakening!

I, on the other hand, have been a yo-yo-dieter since I was a teenager; losing and gaining the same weight – and even more – year after year. I've done everything from starving myself on 1,000 calories a day, to Atkins, shoveling down meat, bacon, cheese and eggs – *I totally cringe today thinking of this*. I lost twenty pounds on the Atkins diet – but my 'sane' internal voice kept nagging me that eating this way was *insane*. I quit Atkins, gained all the weight back, plus some, and turned to Weight Watchers. WW is a great balanced program, but I just couldn't stick with all the measuring and point counting. I wanted to be more 'free' with what I ate. So up and down the weight went for decades. I even went on HCG in 2010. It worked great – but you STARVE! And then, guess what? Right. You gain it back. Again.

When Dr. Jan told Mike he needed to eat an organic vegan diet – I thought since I would be cooking this way for him – I would do it too. I believe this decision has saved my life also. I look and feel younger. I have lots of energy. I lost 30 pounds – and this time – I know I will not gain it back because I have learned how to eat delicious, nutritious, satisfying whole food meals.

Mike and I did not remain strictly vegan. We have lots of vegan meals along with occasional raw, organic cheese and wild caught fish. These days we just accept the house is going to smell like fish when we cook it. So what. We enjoy it, and this 'upgraded' lifestyle of health and nutrition is doing wonders for us in every area of our lives.

> *It is not easy to make major sustainable life-style changes. But it is so worth it!*

- Part Two -

WHY

It's Happening to Everyone

Body Speak!

Chapter 4

WHY We All Need to Change the Way We Eat

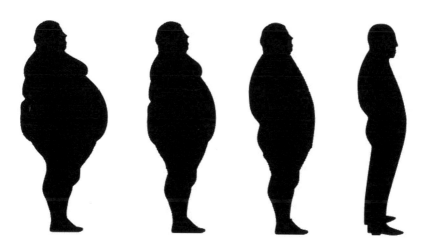

"He who rejects change is the architect of decay. The only human institution which rejects progress is the cemetery,"

Prime Minister Harold Wilson

The Standard American Diet

Some years ago while traveling through Germany, Switzerland and Austria; I was struck by the multitudes of healthy looking people. Everyone, for the most part, looked to be at a good weight and vitality. Good German breakfasts consist of coffee, bread, cheese, and salami – and let's not forget the Germans love their beer and soft, fresh pretzels. What's not to love? Honestly! It was delightful! I marveled how people in Europe are not as obese as we are in America. The heftiest people we saw the entire trip were Americans waddling through the airport terminal going home to the U.S. Something is desperately wrong.

The Standard American Diet – 'SAD' is causing a Health Crisis in our Nation.

SAD is at the root of today's food sensitivities and 'life-style' diseases such as arthritis, obesity, type 2 diabetes, heart disease, kidney failure, infertility, chronic inflammatory disease and cancer. Obesity related disease alone costs the American economy over $150 billion a year.

> # In America, self-afflicted life-style disease is killing more people than contagious disease.

As Americans consume ever increasing amounts of highly processed commercialized foods loaded with sugar, fat, toxic chemicals, pesticides and GMO's; our health and wellbeing is plummeting at alarming rates. While food becomes more manufactured, and 'convenient' – waistlines thicken, health declines and health care costs skyrocket.

Through industrialized agriculture, factory farming, and the manufacturing of chemical laden GMO foods, SAD contains – at best – little to no nutritional value – and at worst is leading multitudes of Americans to early graves. A high price to pay for taste and convenience

FOOD POLITICS

America's toxic food supply is BIG MONEY!

The food industry employs biologists and chemists to enhance food "crave-ability." Meaning, scientists specifically engineer food and drinks people will "crave" and become *addicted* to! The food industry's market shares go up while more and more Americans become addicted to toxically engineered food 'substances' and poisonous drinks.

The tobacco industry learned many years back that curing tobacco leaves with extra sugar *would increase the addiction to cigarettes*. It also greatly increases the instances of lung cancer and heart disease.

Americans crave our chemically engineered drive-thru coffee latté drinks, muffins and donuts, Big Gulp sodas, double-size cheeseburgers, super-sized fries, fried chicken, potato chips, nachos, hot dogs, onion rings, gourmet ice cream, and the list goes on and on.

SAD is taking its toll on Americans – and *sadly* – we now export these fast food franchises to other countries – which are now experiencing a rise in the same chronic diseases rampant in America.

And – what's with all the "energy" drinks flooding the market? These drinks are advertised as "natural" but are anything but! They are loaded with food coloring, fake sugar substitutes and dangerous levels of caffeine. Teenagers are dying out there from consuming too much caffeine within short periods of time.

> *"Last month, a 16-year-old tragically lost his life after consuming an energy drink, a soda and a latte — drinks routinely consumed by and often intensively marketed to youths — all within a few hours. The boy's heart simply couldn't cope with the amount of caffeine in the beverages, according to the coroner."* **Pat Crawford and Wendi Gosliner – Chicago Tribune, May 30, 2017.**

The check-out lines in grocery stores – even Home Depot and mega electronic computer stores – are now accompanied by refrigerators fully stocked with layers of Red Bull, Monster drinks, soda-pop and flavored teas. Cold water? Not so much.

People get so hooked on these sugary, caffeinated beverages they down them all day for energy not realizing these drinks are not only addictive, but they are dehydrating. These poisonous concoctions pump up the heart to dangerous levels and rob the body of vital hydration, causing the 'thirst' to increase and more consumption to occur. "SADLY," *pun intended*, the crave-ability 'experts' have hit their mark! It's all about the almighty dollar with zero concern for the health of humans across the globe.

SAD increases pharmaceutical drug sales as more people suffer from heart burn, acid indigestion, high blood pressure, increased levels of cholesterol and elevated blood sugar. Copious amounts of prescription & over-the-counter drugs are flooding the market claiming to alleviate the symptoms caused by SAD. However, these drugs are made from synthetic chemical ingredients that the body is not equipped to assimilate or utilize. These chemicals build up in the body and cause secondary, serious conditions and illnesses.

> **By using pharmaceuticals to mask Body Speak Symptoms we multiply the negative effects of SAD.**

$$$ Government Subsidies $$$

The Launch of the Fast Food Industry

The federal government subsidizes the production of certain crops; corn, sugar, wheat, soybeans and rice. Government subsidies lead to the over production of these cash crops, causing an imbalance in the marketplace. There are no subsidies for smaller family owned organic farms or for producing the more costly perishable crops, such as fruits and vegetables.

*"The U.S. Department of Agriculture (USDA) spends $25 billion or more a year on **subsidies for farm** businesses. The particular amount each year depends on the market prices of crops and other factors. Most **agricultural subsidies** go to **farmers** of a handful of major crops, including wheat, corn, soybeans, rice, and cotton.*

*Farm subsidies are costly to taxpayers, they distort the economy, and they harm the environment. **Subsidies induce farmers to overproduce, which pushes down prices and creates political demands for more subsidies.** And subsidies hinder farmers from innovating, cutting costs, diversifying their land use, and taking other actions needed to prosper in the competitive global economy"* Agricultural Subsidies | Downsizing the Federal Government Oct 7, 2016
https://www.downsizinggovernment.org/agriculture/subsidies

Thanks to Government subsidies using our hard earned tax dollars the era of industrialized – *cheap* – fast food was born.

These mass produced subsidized crops quickly became the stuff of – white sandwich bread, sugary breakfast cereal, corn chip products, hot dog & hamburger buns, tortillas, pancake mix, high fructose corn syrup – get the idea? These subsidized crops are the basis of the production of fast food and packaged food products.

FOOD VALUE DOLLARS vs HEALTH & QALITY OF FOOD CHOICES

Fast food restaurants – and mid-level food chains, offer a variety of food choices. These products are similarly priced from one fast food chain to the next. After a while they all begin to taste pretty much the same. Some chains are more popular with the kids – say McDonalds for instance. Their advertisements are aimed toward families, and the kid meals and play areas keep consumers coming back for more. I must admit I have purchased kid meals and taken respite in the play area while the kids expend their energy from soda & milk shakes.

There is something to be said about the convenience of fast food that makes it popular with busy families and people on the go. Occasionally, it can serve as a 'treat' on birthdays or after a team sporting event – however, a steady diet of SAD is serving up serious health issues for millions of Americans.

When it comes to appeasing hunger – a $3.99 Big Mac is much more satisfying than a $2.99 cup of iceberg lettuce. When you are hungry and faced with the limited choice between a big, fat juicy hamburger, or a measly cup of limp lettuce – it's a no brainer.

If there were government subsidies for foods like lettuce, tomatoes, cucumbers, avocadoes, seeds, nuts and fruit, then maybe a fast food restaurant would be able to offer customers a better choice – say a luscious, appetizing healthy salad. But there are no subsidies for healthy food choices. Most salads at fast food restaurants are topped with fried chicken, bacon, cheese, croutons, fatty salad dressings, sodium and chemical additives. Again, all manufactured with subsidized tax dollars. And that unhealthy salad – in some fast food chains costs more than a super-sized burger meal!

Of course – we are talking here about spending dollars, and food politics – not healthy food choices. The SAD truth is – Americans want and *crave* fatty fried food, sugary soda, candy, sweets and junk food. Most Americans going out to eat are not counting calories or looking for healthy food choices. Some are, and things are beginning to change, but for the most part people want what they want – when they want it! Right now – and affordable!

According to the *Consumer Reports Fast Food Buying Guide* – people are more interested in how far their food dollars will stretch – rather than the quality of food or the amount of calories in their food;

> *"Most diners aren't concerned about dieting when they eat out. Only 20 percent of survey respondents consider the availability of healthy menu options when choosing a restaurant. And just 19 percent of readers admitted to ordering a healthy meal during their most recent dining experience. Women were more conscientious than men. Forty-two percent (vs. 28 percent of men surveyed) ordered lower-calorie fare from restaurants that conspicuously displayed nutritional information on the menu. Most people, though, don't notice such information. **When we asked respondents if their menus displayed calorie and fat counts, 51 percent said they were unsure,"** (author emphasis). http://www.consumerreports.org/cro/fast-food-restaurants/buying-guide.htm*

According to Consumer Reports 51% of the people they surveyed are not even aware of menus displaying the calorie counts of food. This is an indication that over half of America is not interested in health or calories when eating out.

Personally, I've been out with family and friends who do make intentional decisions based on calorie counts in menus. In fact, my son Ben was horrified when his favorite restaurant updated their menu to include calorie counts. The number was shocking and it helped him to let go of a few of his fatty favorites and make healthier choices. We will talk more about calories a little later on because counting calories is not necessary when making the right food choices.

WE DON'T WANT A "NANNY STATE!"

The derogatory term – Nanny State – is becoming a popular identifier for critics who oppose policies for food labeling and portion size.

The accusation of becoming a 'Nancy State' is bandied about in political circles – and in the main stream media – to criticize and oppose all perceived 'interference' by law makers to enforce things like mandatory food labeling laws, portion size, and soft drinks sold in school cafeterias.

When New York City Mayor Michael Bloomberg proposed in May 2012, that soft drinks sold in public venues, restaurants and sidewalk carts should be limited to 16 ounces – the soft-drink industry fought back by launching a vicious NANNY STATE smear campaign against him.

In an article published by Legal Insurrection on June 3, 2012, a photograph created by ConsumerFreedom.com was used to portray Mayor Bloomberg as **The Nanny**, wearing a blue nanny dress;

> *"You only thought you lived in the land of the free. New Yorkers need a Mayor, not a Nanny."*

> *"**Bye Bye Venti** – Nanny Bloomberg has taken his strange obsession with what you eat one step further. He now wants to make it illegal to serve "sugary drinks" bigger than 16 oz. What's next? Limits on the width of a pizza slice, size of a hamburger or amount of cream cheese on your bagel"* http://legalinsurrection.com/2012/06/the-nanny/

Americans do not like being controlled, censored, or told what they can eat and drink. All is fair out there in 'Big Gulp' double-double cheeseburger land. After all, it's a free country and people have the right to enjoy their food and beverages. I agree, freedom is a wonderful thing, and I do not want the government telling me how much cream cheese to put on my bagel!

However, some laws and policies are quite helpful and necessary because no one thrives in chaos and lawlessness. Kids need Nannies. Adults benefit from self-control and sensible food choices. A balance must be found somewhere in the sane middle.

In the land of the free and the home of the brave – 'sanity' needs to prevail before everyone ends up diving off the cliff of obesity life-style choices and ending up dead like a bunch of mindless, fat, diseased lemmings.

In the words of Oliver Wendell Holms, "Your right to harm yourself stops when I have to pay for it!"

The soft drink industry does not want any regulations on the size of their products. Mayor Bloomberg was only suggesting limiting a single soda to 16 ounces. There is NOTHING restricting the number of single portions sold to a consumer, just the *size* of what is considered a *single* portion.

It's all about market share. The fact is – any kind of regulation of sugary drinks cuts into the profits of the soda industry. And let's face it – they have the money to fight back in advertising and have no qualms about using defaming and exaggerated smear campaigns against anyone who threatens their profits.

Freedom is not actually free. There is always a price to pay along the way for living in excess and toxic food overload. The reality is even if the human brain chooses to consciously ignore the ramifications of eating a diet full of fatty, sugary, toxic food, the body does *not*. The body keeps score. This magnificent bio-machine keeps track of every molecule of every substance that enters it. And, the body functions to keep us alive at all costs. It does the best it can, but there is no escape from the long term effects of the bombardment of a constant diet of SAD. Yes, we are free to indulge – but at what cost?

> **One in three Americans will receive a cancer diagnosis in their lifetime. Chronic auto-immune diseases are rising at alarming rates. According to *Medical News Today*, heart disease is now the number one cause of death in *both* men and women. The rates of childhood obesity and cancer have caused scientists to predict that this present generation of children is expected to experience a lower life expectancy than their parents.**

You've probably heard it said in the 'beauty' and 'anti-aging' industry that 50 is the new 30 – but I say that in the area of health and nutrition, SAD and the toxic world we live in are causing the 50's & 60's to become the new 80's.

It's time to become informed, take action in our own life – and take our health back.

Chapter 5

The Misinformation Wars!

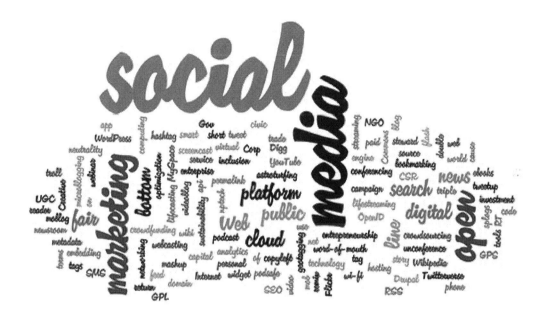

The HEALTH INDUSTRY is *BIG BUSINESS*! FOOD and BEVERAGE is *BIG BUSINESS* – Big Business wants your money, and does not care about your health. So BUYER BEWARE! Be your own health advocate and don't believe what you see at face value.

Traversing the "WWW" Highway of Truth, Misinformation & Propaganda

When our Naturopath doctor told Mike to STOP EATING SUGAR – because sugar feeds cancer – this was the first time we had ever heard such a thing. Really? Could this be true? It must be true, Dr. Jan told us so. We took her statement at face value because we trust her and she has a long history of healing people. Both Mike and I cut out all sugar because of Dr. Jan's warning.

Dr. Jan also sent us website links to help get us started on the journey of understanding health and nutrition. I checked out every link she emailed, which launched me into deeper understanding and continued research into alternative healing measures. I heard about the damaging effects of sugar and how it feeds cancer from these functional medicine doctors and naturopathic healers.

At that time Mike's brother was battling cancer too, and we shared this information about sugar feeding cancer with him. We desperately wanted him to embark on the same road we were on to try to arrest the spread of his cancer and prolong his life.

Sadly, his daughter did a search on the internet to find out if this claim about sugar was true and later told me she found *nothing* on the web confirming this statement. I was flummoxed because I had seen it first hand through my own research. I didn't understand how my niece had not seen this information – to me it was easy to find.

However, it was only easy to find because our doctor had already sent us direct links to the right sources. After what my niece told me, I did my own Google search asking, *"Does sugar feed cancer?"* and I saw why my niece had so much trouble finding out the truth. Sugar industry advertisements and misinformation came up first in the search prompts. If you really wanted to find the answer to this question you had to push past the first few pages of misleading, diversionary tactics and misdirection.

I am happy to report that today, the truth about sugar and cancer is much more readily available in search engines. In fact, here is a great source that comes up now on the first page: http://beatcancer.org/blog-posts/5-reasons-cancer-and-sugar-are-best-friends/

> **The reason I am sharing this story with you is to warn you – or rather *remind* you as you traverse this journey toward health and nutrition, that there is a real war out there for your mind, your food beliefs and your food spending dollars. And advertisers lie.**

Who doesn't LOVE the modern age of instant, endless information? I certainly do.

When I was a kid the arrival of the latest edition of the Encyclopedia Britannica sent me into a passion of knowledge hungry bliss. Just cracking open the glorious leather bound treasure and smelling the delicious aroma of freshly minted pages of information ignited my soul. I would flip through the colorful volume lush with fascinating discovery and hold the book to my chest wishing with my entire young heart that somehow all this wonderful knowledge would magically infuse itself into my brain with perfect memory and comprehension. Wow, I would be so smart I mused, probably smarter than anyone else in the whole wide world if I had this much knowledge inside of my head.

There Was a Time the Printed Word Could be Trusted

For over a century the Encyclopedia Britannica was one of the world's leading publishers of scholarly based, factual, information. They were trusted, because they were trustworthy. There was a time the printed word could be trusted. If it appeared in a book, or on television, or in a newspaper, Americans were safe to believe the information. Back in those days' people never suspected the world of information and knowledge would morph into the sea of tangled, confusing and purposeful misinformation that it is today.

To successfully navigate through the controversial world of health and nutrition we need to take a brief look at where modern day belief systems over food and nutrition come from. And to do this – we start by following the money.

FOOD FIGHT – DUCK & COVER!

We've all seen those ridiculous food fights in the movies. One character decides to launch a whip cream pie at another character igniting the entire room of diners into a full blown food throwing frenzy.

Food fights may get a chuckle or two in the moves – but they are far from funny in real life. Little do people realize, they are caught in the middle of the vicious, nasty, lying, manipulating Wall Street competition for America's food spending dollars.

Marketing Dollars – Weapons in the Food Fight

People trust what they see on TV ads and commercials. Honestly, in this day and age of misinformation – believing in advertising is akin to believing cartoons are real life. The food industry goes to extremes to influence what people think about food. The industry hires brilliant marketing manipulators to foist their wares on the gullible public.

The meat and dairy council work hard to make people believe their bodies are made stronger from the calcium in milk and the protein in beef. This is not true, and we'll see why later on in the Protein Controversy chapter.

When elevated cholesterol levels began to rise from the over consumption of beef and dairy, the 'beef council' vilified eggs as the cholesterol raising culprit. In order to combat this attack the 'egg council' launched their own campaign of – *"The Incredible Edible Egg,"* which helped to boost their profit shares after the beef council's nasty attack.

And let's not forget what the egg council did when those pesky vegans dared to create a popular egg-free mayo!

> *"With its egg-free recipe, Just Mayo had become a darling of vegans, a hot investment for Silicon Valley venture capitalists and an avatar for alternatives to industrial agriculture.*

> *"But to the nation's $7-billion egg industry, Just Mayo posed an existential crisis so serious that a federally supervised trade group launched a*

secret two-year campaign to thwart the San Francisco start-up that makes it.

"The campaign against Beyond Eggs, the original name of company behind Just Mayo, included flirting with an offer from a consultant who bragged he could rid the product from <u>Whole Foods</u>' shelves "with one phone call," and jokes among American Egg Board members and affiliates about "pooling our money to put a hit" on the company's founder, emails show."

"The investigation, sparked by documents obtained through the <u>Freedom of Information Act</u> by a Massachusetts Institute of Technology researcher and his Washington attorney, reveals the lengths the American Egg Board appeared willing to go to crush Just Mayo, its manufacturer, now called Hampton Creek, and the firm's founder, Josh Tetrick." <u>http://www.latimes.com/business/la-fi-egg-board-investigation-20161007-snap-story.html</u>

Let's Take Soy For Instance…*(out of our lives!)*

The food fight over soy is fierce in the misinformation war.

When soy first hit the market it was touted as the 'cure all' for what ailed you. After all just look at the Asians, consuming oodles of soy and noodles while looking young and living longer than most other cultures in today's world.

However… once again – I have to say it – **SOY is *BIG BUSINESS*!** The slightest positive result from one limited test study is exploited by the soy council and exaggerated to the point of lunacy. Even suggesting soy be injected in utero to female embryos in order to reduce the risk of developing breast cancer! Come on – *for real*? I trust you will agree this is utter madness.

First of all, Asians do not consume as much soy as the industry claims. And the soy traditionally consumed for centuries is fermented, which makes it easier to digest. For the most part, soy was considered to be a poor folk food, and grown in

Body Speak!

order to fertilize the soil, not be consumed in mass quantities. Livestock doesn't even care to graze on the remains of a soy crop.

> **The soy industry claims multiple health benefits from eating soy, but true scientific research now indicates that soy is adding to illness in America, not decreasing it.**

The Mayo Clinic evaluated and graded the evidence allegedly supporting thirty-seven health claims of the soy industry. The grading system went from A – F.

"A" Signifies strong scientific evidence,

"B" Good,

"C" Unclear, more scientific tests required,

"F" Strong scientific evidence against this use.

The Mayo Clinic assigned two A's, two B's, thirty-two C's and one F.

Out of thirty-seven health benefit claims The Mayo Clinic allotted only two "A's" the first being the fact that soy has protein and is approved for dietary use. The second was claiming it lowers cholesterol. However, the studies showing soy lowered cholesterol worked best in people who substituted soy for *all animal protein*.

Guess what happens when a person removes all animal protein from their diet? If you guessed it would lower cholesterol then you are right! It isn't the soy that decreases cholesterol – **it's the removal of animal food that lowers cholesterol**.

Even the two "B's" allotted suggested that more research is necessary – and the thirty-two "C's" all stated specifically that more science is necessary to prove this claim.

The one "F" was allotted for the claim soy helps with osteoporosis.

You can read the full article here if you are interested;
http://www.mayoclinic.org/drugs-supplements/soy/evidence/hrb-20060012

Here is what Dr. Mercola, orthopedic surgeon and leading voice in reliable health and nutrition information has to say about the dangers of soy:

Soy Dangers Summarized by Dr. Mercola

1. High levels of phytic acid in soy reduce assimilation of calcium, magnesium, copper, iron and zinc. Phytic acid in soy is not neutralized by ordinary preparation methods such as soaking, sprouting, and long, slow cooking, but only with long fermentation. High-phytic diets have caused growth problems in children.

2. Trypsin inhibitors in soy interfere with protein digestion and may cause pancreatic disorders. In test animals, soy containing trypsin inhibitors caused stunted growth.

3. Soy phytoestrogens disrupt endocrine function and have the potential to cause infertility and to promote breast cancer in adult women.

4. Soy phytoestrogens are potent anti-thyroid agents that cause hypothyroidism and may cause thyroid cancer. In infants, consumption of soy formula has been linked to autoimmune thyroid disease.

5. Vitamin B12 analogs in soy are not absorbed and actually increase the body's requirement for B12.

6. Soy foods increase the body's requirement for Vitamin D. Toxic synthetic Vitamin D2 is added to soy milk.

7. Fragile proteins are over-denatured during high temperature processing to make soy protein isolate and textured vegetable protein.

8. Processing of soy protein results in the formation of toxic lysinoalanine and highly carcinogenic nitrosamines.

9. Free glutamic acid or MSG, a potent neurotoxin, is formed during soy food processing and additional amounts are added to many soy foods to mask soy's unpleasant taste.

10. Soy foods contain high levels of aluminum, which is toxic to the nervous system and the kidneys.

http://articles.mercola.com/sites/articles/archive/2010/12/04/soy-dangers-summarized.aspx

The examples I've shared here are only the tip of the iceberg. The misinformation wars rage all around us all the time.

In this instant age of technology, social media and YouTube, people become famous – just for being famous! Being popular or famous is not a credential for trustworthiness.

Personally, I do not trust advertising of any kind. I record the TV shows I like so that I can fast forward through the commercials. I navigate the maze of the misinformation highway by choosing to listen to people who have long track records of actually healing people. When I find a professional I trust, I read their material and listen to their lectures and buy their books. I have to say here though, if that person's news letters and emails turn into a barrage of Ad campaigns for their latest product – I tend to stop listening to them. I feel when a person becomes all about their product they too can tend to become all about the money, and not all about the health.

Chapter 6

The World is a Dangerous Place Pesticides, Environmental Toxins, GMO's & Factory Farming

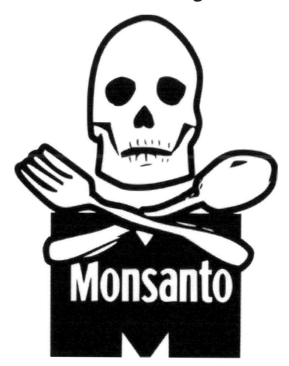

Modern technology and the advancement of industrialization have benefitted the world in many wonderful and exciting ways. At the same time, it has polluted the earth and created toxins that cause cancer and are destroying the planet.

Where do all the waste products from factories and manufacturing facilities end up? In the ground, in the oceans, in our drinking water – and you guessed it – in our bodies!

THE DANGERS OF PESTICIDES

Pesticides & Cancer

In the US, one of every two men and one of every three women are likely to develop cancer over the course of a lifetime – and pesticides are part of the reason why.

The American Cancer Society estimated in 2015 that nearly 1.7 million people would be diagnosed with cancer. Some cancers are on the rise, including childhood cancers, leukemia and testicular cancer. We are experiencing a cancer epidemic, and evidence is growing ever stronger that pesticide exposure is a key factor to this alarming trend.

Chemicals can trigger cancer in a variety of ways, including disrupting hormones, damaging DNA, inflaming tissues and turning genes on or off. Many pesticides are "known or probable" carcinogens.

Children are especially at risk of developing cancer from pesticide exposure. Studies show that pesticide exposure during pregnancy and throughout childhood increases the risk of cancer among children. Girls who were exposed to DDT before they reach puberty were found to be five times more likely to develop breast cancer in middle age.

Pesticides & Infertility

Infertility is becoming more common among young adults, both male and female. One of the contributing factors has been linked to the proliferation of pesticides.

Many pesticides and industrial chemicals are capable of interfering with the proper functioning of estrogen, androgen (male sex hormone) and thyroid hormones in humans and animals. These substances are called endocrine disruptors. Exposure can cause sterility or decreased fertility, impaired development, birth defects of the reproductive tract and metabolic disorders.

INDUSTRIAL CHEMICAL INVASION – *BIOSLUDGE!*

In 2004, Jack Black and Ben Stiller were in a movie called Envy. Jack Black invented a poop vaporizing aerosol spray called; *Vapoorize.* All you needed to do was spray Vapoorize on the dog, horse or cat poop in your yard and it vanished! No one knew where the poop actually went – but they didn't really care – out of sight out of mind, right? The Vapoorize flew off the shelves making Jack Black a wealthy man. Later on in the plot we discover the vaporized poop has liquefied into a harmful chemical and seeped into the ground, killing a prized race horse that ate apples from a tree that had soaked up toxins from the soil.

WHERE *DOES* THE POOP GO?

Have you heard of biosolids? It is something like Vapoorize! A toxic blend of human excrement and chemicals.

All the waste from every city is collected, separated from water, composted, and then spread on rural farms that grow foods. This substance is called "biosolids." There are many sewage recycling centers for biosolids.

Here is how the Environmental Protective Agency (EPA) defines biosolids:

> *"What are* **Biosolids***? They are nutrient-rich organic materials resulting from the treatment of domestic sewage in a treatment facility. When treated and processed, these residuals can be recycled and applied as fertilizer to improve and maintain productive soils and stimulate plant growth."*

If the EPA says biosolids are used to improve and maintain productive soil, then it must be true, right? Wrong.

According to Mike Adams – the Health Ranger – investigative food reporter, and forensic food scientist, the EPA has been covering up the truth about the mass chemical poisoning of America. Toxic and cancer causing industrial waste of heavy metals, human excrement, pharmaceutical, and veterinary waste are being made into fertilizer and being dumped on farm lands.

Mike Adams, the Health Ranger claims "Biosludge" is the greatest environmental crime in America.

Here's how it goes, rural farms are offered "free" *organic* fertilizer from a nearby city. They claim it is part of an "agricultural support program" – and large trucks bring loads of material and dump it onto the farmland. This load of 'crap' smells horrendous as it off gasses toxic odors that continue for weeks before dissipating.

And then the farmer's families begin to become ill from mysterious diseases...Hmm... think there may be a connection...? Seems like a no brainer to me! But these farmers are intentionally lied to, and believe the free soil is harmless, and actually a "gift" to help them. So why would they suspect they are sick from the toxic fertilizer? It's time they figured it out.

Mike Adams tested the "Free Fertilizer" of three companies; Dillo Dirt from Austin Texas, Milorganite from Milwaukee and Organic Sound Gro ("The Dirty Gardener").

Here is what Mike Adam's at CWC Labs found when he tested the biosolids:

- Concentrated human feces; human waste from city recycled into 'green' product
- Industrial waste from US cities
- Analysis shows heavy metals; lead, mercury, arsenic, copper plus nickel, molybdenum and cadmium
- 300 – 550 chemicals such as pesticides, toxins, veterinary drugs, nervous system drugs, stimulants, and antibiotics

This toxic biosludge is sold to consumers for use on home gardens – that means you and me. I've wondered why some bags of fertilizer say – *"Do not use on edible plants."* Now I know why, because *they know* it is a poisonous carcinogenic nightmare. And now you know too!

BUYER beware – when you are purchasing fertilizer, look on the bottom of the bag for cancer warnings!

CANCER IS NOT INEVITABLE

The Misunderstood Connection Between Genes and Cancer

Everyone's DNA is made up of genes. Genes are a portion of a DNA molecule that serves as the basic unit of heredity. These are particular characteristics of heredity passed along from a parent to a child that determine things like height, hair and skin color and region of origin.

> ### It's been said, "Genes load the gun, but the environment pulls the trigger." Possessing a certain gene – does NOT mean you will get cancer.

As previously discussed, Western Medicine believes genes are the determining factor of whether or not someone develops cancer, along with some environmental carcinogens.

There are specific genes that cause people to be more susceptible to developing certain types of cancer. You can think of these genes as having a "predisposition" toward developing cancer. However, possessing these genes does not mean you will develop cancer.

The media hysteria over Angelina Jolie's discovery of the BRCA1 / BRCA2 breast cancer gene, and her subsequent decision to remove both of her healthy breasts, became front page news. Two years later she had her healthy ovaries and fallopian tubes removed. Angelina was concerned because breast cancer runs in her family so when the gene was discovered – she chose the RADICAL solution of removing her healthy female body parts.

Many people believe Angelina was incredibly brave to make such a drastic and bold decision. It was her body, and her decision to make. She sought help from people who believe the theory that genes are the sole cause of cancer and she took their advice. If she wasn't convinced she was in serious danger, she never would have proceeded with these drastic surgeries BEFORE cancer developed.

BUT… was it bravery? Or was it fear and misinformation?

The reality is – gene detection technology is relatively new and not a perfect science. At first, scientists believed the human body consisted of 100,000 genes. Today, it is estimated the human genome consists of approximately 24,000 genes. New discoveries build on older discoveries as technology advances.

According to Sunil Pai MD, author of *An Inflammation Nation,*

> *"Only around 2 percent of women with breast cancer test positive for BRCA markers. Among those who have these markers, there's only (at most) a 30 percent chance that the gene will express itself. That means that most women (98 percent) would not test positive for BRCA1 or BRCA2, and those who did would have a 70 percent chance that the gene would never express."*

Dr. Pai goes on to explain the true instigators behind the media blitz touting the benefits of discovering the BRCA1 / BRCA2 gene marker. It was a company trying to patent a $15,000 test to determine if a person has this gene. This company stood to earn hundreds of millions of dollars in a very short time. The U.S. Supreme Court blocked the patent, reducing the test cost, but its utility is still very low.

In reality, there are over 500 different genes that have been shown to increase the risk of developing breast cancer. Scientists have discovered about 250,000 possible gene combinations for breast cancer. Testing for only two genes (BRCA1 / BRCA2) does not adequately establish risk.

> *"The BRCA gene scare was really quite a Hollywood hype, and I'm not judging her. She saw her Mother die a very horrible death, but there was a lot of mis-information. The BRCA genes are actually cancer-protective genes. They help to repair DNA damage, so the BRCA gene, if it mutates, then it can cause a problem possibly, but what causes it to mutate? Look at the foods. Look at the radiation, BRCA genes are tumor suppressive protective genes,"*
> Dr. Veronique Desaulniers, The Truth About Cancer, A Global Quest.

As a woman, there is always an underlying fear your breasts will "betray you" and one day develop cancer. The breast cancer industry has done an excellent job of making women feel like their breasts are unstable, volatile, unpredictable, and apparently, dangerous body parts that can one day rise up and kill you! So you had better find this gene, and then cut your breasts off – just to be sure. It's monstrous and barbaric in my opinion.

With thousands of possible genetic cancer risk combinations, even the best genetic testing can only indicate a *potential* cancer risk. Having a genetic risk factor does not mean you will get cancer. Furthermore, it is impossible and impractical to avoid every possible genetic risk. So what can we do to minimize our cancer risk? Epigenetics to the rescue!

> **Epigenetics - Is the scientific understanding that genes in the body are switched on or off through various means including diet, lifestyle and environment.**

Epigenetics and Cancer

Genes comprising our genetic risk factors have switches that can be turned on or off. The major factors influencing these switches are diet and lifestyle, things within our control. This is both good and bad. As can be seen from the present cancer epidemic, SAD activates the gene switches toward the development of cancer and other serious illnesses.

Taking personal responsibility for our health by leaving SAD behind and incorporating whole foods, detoxification, stress management, exercise and natural holistic therapies helps keep genetic risk factors dormant. In fact, we can actually change the expression of our genes from *risk factor markers* to *protective factor markers* by choosing a healthy lifestyle.

GENETICALLY MODIFIED ORGANISMS (GMO'S)

Up until 2013, I had no idea GMO's existed. I was discussing natural hormone replacement therapy with my functional medicine doctor who did not have time to tell me exactly what GMO's are – but she warned me to stop eating them – especially corn tortillas! Yikes! I was clueless that eating corn tortillas posed a hazard to my health.

I was intrigued by this and began to search labels for GMO products. This is easier said than done, however, as the labeling of GMO's is fiercely contended in the political arena in both America and Canada. Advocates for labeling GMO products have been battling in the U.S. court system for years – and as of the writing of this book, August, 2017, there are no laws in place requiring the labeling of GMO products in the United States.

According to the Non-GMO Project Organization, sixty-four countries around the world, including Australia, Japan, and all of the countries in the European Union, require genetically modified foods to be labelled. While a 2015 NBC survey found that 93% of Americans believe genetically modified foods should be labelled, GMO's are not required to be labelled in the U.S. and Canada.

Food politics at work – "He with the most money wins."

What is a GMO?

A GMO is a genetically modified organism of a plant, animal, microorganism or other organism whose genetic makeup has been modified by using genetic material resulting from the splicing of DNA fragments. This relatively new science, known as transgenic technology, creates unstable combinations of plant, animal, bacterial and viral genes that DO NOT OCCUR in nature or through traditional crossbreeding methods.

The idea of genetic modification in itself is not necessarily a bad thing. Gene splicing technology enables scientists to isolate a particular favorable attribute in one gene and then combine that gene with other isolated genes to create something that did not exist before.

One of the positive claims of the GMO manufacturers is that gene technology helps extend the shelf life of GMO produce. So the goal of the new Arctic Golden Delicious GMO apple – arriving this fall in supermarkets in the U.S. - is to tolerate a longer shelf life without turning brown.

It is perfectly normal for apples to turn brown soon after cutting them and there are no harmful side effects from eating a slightly brown apple. But – a nice package of sliced apples wrapped pretty in the grocery store that does not brown is a sales gimmick. It might look prettier – but it is far from nutritious, and in fact is dangerous to your health – *because* – GMO's are engineered to withstand copious amounts of pesticides and the herbicide glyphosate, and not die. I will explain more about this deadly combination a little farther on.

GMO's A Global Hungry Conglomerate

GMO seeds are engineered by six major corporations the "Big 6" are; BASF, Bayer, DuPont, Dow Chemical Company, Monsanto and Syngenta. These corporations dominate the agricultural input market – that is, they own the world's seed, pesticide and biotechnology industries. These companies seek to patent and control the global food supply.

Recently the German based drug company Bayer purchased Monsanto for a whopping $66 Billion. This positions Bayer at the top of the leader board controlling approximately one fourth of the planet's seed market.

> **The U.S. and Canadian governments have approved GMO's based on studies conducted by the SAME CORPORATIONS who created them and profit from their sales.**

Are GMO's Safe?

The world's largest chemical companies claim they are! The rest of the world is not convinced.

Most developed nations do not consider GMO's to be safe and have put significant restrictions, and in some cases, outright bans, on the production and sale of GMO's.

There are no long-term – independent – scientific studies to determine the safety of GMO products. And get this one – there is NO FDA requirement for peer reviewed, independent studies. Zero. None. What a racket!

No FDA GMO Testing Required

The GMO manufacturers claim genetically modified foods are perfectly safe – however – *this is based on their own internal reviews*.

> *"FDA does not itself test whether genetically engineered foods are safe. The FDA has repeatedly made this clear. As Jason Dietz, a policy analyst at FDA explains about genetically engineered food: "It's the manufacturer's responsibility to insure that the product is safe." Or, as FDA spokesperson Theresa Eisenman said, "it is the manufacturer's responsibility to ensure that the [GMO] food products it offers for sale are safe…"*

> *"Nor does the FDA require independent pre-market safety testing for genetically engineered food. As a matter of practice, **the agrichemical companies submit their own studies to the FDA as part of a voluntary "consultation." Moreover, the FDA does not require the companies to submit full and complete information about these studies.** Rather, as the FDA has testified, "After the studies are completed, a summary of the data and information on the safety and nutritional assessment are provided to the FDA for review." https://usrtk.org/the-fda-does-not-test-whether-gmos-are-safe*

In the words of my dearly departed Grandpa – believing the chemical companies and GMO manufacturers claiming their products are safe based on their own internal studies is like – "hiring the fox to watch the henhouse!" There are zero regulatory measures in place to actually guarantee the safety of these products.

Monsanto GMO Bt-Corn *Itself* is a Pesticide!

Bt-corn is designed to actually BECOME the poison *itself* when the insect eats the corn its stomach explodes.
Bt-corn is a bio-toxin; a biologically engineered poison that is saturating the food supply.

Monsanto isolated a particular gene from soil bacteria called Bt (Bacillus thuringiensis) that breaks open the stomach of certain insects and kills them.

Alarming reports are surfacing that Bt-toxin has been identified in the blood of both pregnant and non-pregnant women, as well as the umbilical blood of their babies. It has been determined that the consumption of Bt-foods is the source of this pollution in the blood.

It is bad enough to spray poison "on" corn – it is a different thing entirely to make the *corn itself into poison!* If Bt-corn causes the stomach of insects to explode, what do you think it does to the guts of the humans who eat it? In time it destroys gut villi and protective tissue and leads to multitudes of food sensitivities, degenerative and autoimmune diseases.

GMO corn and soy are the foundation of all fast food and packaged food products. GMO Canola oil, soybean oil and high fructose corn-syrup are used to cook and flavor foods such as the delectable deep fried donuts we love and those delicious chips at Mexican restaurants. Which unfortunately, sums up the tastiest components of SAD to perfection.

What are the impacts of GMO's on the environment?

More than 80% of all GMO crops grown worldwide are engineered for herbicide tolerance. This mean the plants stay alive despite being doused with profuse amounts of toxic herbicides like Roundup.

GMO crops are responsible for the abundance of herbicide resistant "super weeds" and "super bugs."

"Super-Bugs:" Bt corn, which accounts for 65 percent of all corn grown in the U.S., has produced a new generation of insects resistant to the built-in pesticide within the plants.

"Super-Weeds:" Bt corn is generating the rapid emergence of super-weeds resistant to glyphosate.

> *http://www.huffingtonpost.com/dr-mercola/bt-corn_b_2442072.html*

> http://articles.mercola.com/sites/articles/archive/2012/05/29/genetically-modified-crops-insects-emerged.aspx

Nature has a way of fighting back, so now more and more toxic chemicals are required to grow GMO crops. The use of chemicals like 2,4D, a major component of Agent Orange, are increasing. Of course it is the chemical companies who manufacture these GMO seeds – so if more poison is needed to kill super weeds and super bugs, it simply means more profit for them. Win, win is their motto. People becoming ill and dying of cancer is no concern of theirs.

GMO *'TERMINATOR'* Seeds Do Not Reproduce!

> **GMO manufacturers claim their seeds are the best thing there is for stopping world hunger. But if these seeds must be produced in secret laboratories of patent protected companies, and these seeds DO NOT REPRODUCE how is this sustainable for anything other than the sustained profit of multi-billion dollar chemical conglomerates?**

GMO's are patented seeds – engineered specifically not to reproduce – forcing farmers to buy new seeds each growing season. This is very expensive for farmers. Traditionally seeds are reserved from each harvest to be used in the next planting season. Purposely designing seeds that do not reproduce is a deliberate ploy to keep farmers enslaved to the GMO seed monopoly.

Farmers who choose not to grow GMO crops are in big trouble if GMO seeds are carried on the wind from miles away and happen to be found growing in their fields. Company men peruse the farm lands enforcing patent laws which incur extreme penalties and lawsuits for farmers. Many family farms have been driven out of business by heartless corporations creating amalgamations of engineered seeds in an effort to obtain global dominance of all agriculture on the planet.

GMO's & Roundup-Ready - Glyphosate

Glyphosate is the patented herbicide in Roundup. This herbicide destroys the body's natural gut microbiome; particularly the beneficial enzyme, transglutaminase. This enzyme performs many roles in the body including fertilization, reproduction, and blood clotting.

According to Mike Adams of Natural News:

"Glyphosate is actually the world's most-used herbicide, and is used on more than 175 million acres of land just in the United States.

General Mills' Cheerios, perhaps one of our nation's most ubiquitous and iconic cereals, was found to contain a whopping 1,125.3 ppb of glyphosate residue. Ritz crackers contained just over 270 ppb of the herbicide. More shocking, perhaps, was the amount of glyphosate found in a Kashi product. Kashi is often seen as a "health food" brand, but their soft-baked oatmeal dark chocolate cookies contained more glyphosate residue than Ritz crackers, at just over 275 ppb. Glyphosate is even used on non-GM crops as a way to dry them out and speed up the harvesting process. The pervasiveness of this toxic herbicide is almost astounding." http://www.naturalnews.com/056152_glyphosate_food_contamination_weed_killer.html#ixzz4UYaXlGHH

Glyphosate Clings to Toxic Metals

Glyphosate acts as a "metal chelator" that clings to toxic metals flowing through the bloodstream such as mercury, aluminum and arsenic. In fact, it 'hides' itself in such a way, clinging to arsenic, that the arsenic is not 'detected' by the body's defense mechanisms until it gets into the kidneys where it lets loose and floods the kidneys with a blast of undiluted arsenic.

Dr. Stephanie Seneff, Senior Research Scientist at the MIT Computer Science and Artificial Intelligence Laboratory has conducted several peer reviewed scientific studies on the effect of glyphosate on humans;

"Glyphosate is possibly the most important factor in the development of multiple chronic diseases and conditions that have become prevalent in Westernized societies," including but not limited to:

"Autism, Alzheimer's, ALS, allergies, gastrointestinal diseases such as inflammatory bowel disease, chronic diarrhea, colitis and Crohn's disease, cardiovascular disease, cancer, infertility, depression, obesity, Parkinson's

disease, Multiple sclerosis, and more;" Dr. Stephanie Seneff – Vaccines, Autism and Glyphosate; http://vaccine-injury.info/gmo-autism-link.cfm

Glyphosate & Gluten

Glyphosate reduces Lactobacillus (good gut bacteria) which leads to impaired digestion.

Glyphosate attaches to the gluten molecule and essentially, "mimics" gluten, therein tricking the body to react to gluten as if it is was a dangerous intruder.

> **Gluten, the innocent protein substance of wheat – eaten by humans for millennium – is now perceived by the body to be a 'toxic' substance it must attack, causing autoimmune disorders which are now referred to as 'Leaky Gut.'**

Leaky Gut Syndrome

Today, Americans face a near epidemic of bowel related indigestion illnesses. Independent scientific studies are finding links between glyphosate and serious illness including cell death, birth defects, miscarriage, low sperm counts, DNA damage, and more recently a syndrome known as; 'Leaky Gut.'

When the intestinal villi are damaged, small 'leaks' occur in the intestines which cause undigested food particles and undiluted toxins to enter the blood stream prematurely, bypassing the full breakdown process.

Here is an easy to understand definition of Leaky Gut from the creators of the website; Specific Carbohydrate Diet (SCD).

"The term Leaky Gut Syndrome is used to describe the condition of "Hyper Permeable Intestines," a fancy medical term that means the intestinal lining

has become more porous, with more holes developing that are larger in size and the screening out process is no longer functioning properly. The fallout results in larger, undigested food molecules and other "bad stuff" (yeast, toxins, and all other forms of waste) that your body normally doesn't allow through, to flow freely into your bloodstream," http://scdlifestyle.com/2010/03/the-scd-diet-and-leaky-gut-syndrome/

Basically, Leaky Gut is the destruction of the protective lining of the gut.

GLYPHOSATE Destroys Good Gut Bacteria

Not only does Glyphosate destroy the protective lining of the gut – it destroys good bacteria necessary for the body's immune system to fight germs and disease.

Leaky Gut contributes to inflammation markers in the body, causing the body to send off an immune response to attack good bacteria, igniting an autoimmune response which can lead to diseases like Crohn's, colitis and irritable bowel diseases, among many others.

A leaky gut releases toxins directly into the bloodstream and puts a HUGE strain on the liver. The body literally goes to war against these intruders, which causes inflammation throughout the entire body. The body does not know precisely 'what' to attack so unfortunately it begins to attack *itself* – and this is what is known as an 'autoimmune' disorder; when the body goes into hyper 'immune' response against its own flesh.

Celiac Disease

Celiac disease is an autoimmune illness affecting primarily the small intestine that occurs in people who are genetically predisposed. Meaning; celiac disease is something you are born with. It is usually difficult to isolate because the symptoms of celiac disease are wide reaching and can affect everything from poor digestion to mental illness.

Celiac disease is worsened by eating wheat because the gluten protein molecule in wheat is difficult to digest. For these people, when gluten is eaten the body treats it is an enemy 'invader' that must be destroyed. The body goes into hyper alert and destroys the inner lining of the small intestine and damages the villi. The more damaged the villi become, the less nutrients are absorbed from the food we eat, and the more susceptible we become to airborne illnesses because the body's immune system is compromised.

A weak immune system contributes to the formation of cancer cells because the body is flooded with toxins and unable to isolate and destroy the carcinogenic free radicals moving through the blood stream.

The Lymph System

The lymph system is the body's sewer system, designed to rid the body of all toxins and unnecessary waste. The lymph system helps 'analyze' foreign substances and creates powerful antibodies and white blood cells that kill viruses, harmful bacteria and cancer cells and then removes them from the body.

It is vital that the lymph system remains functioning and flushing the body of waste products continuously. If the lymph system backs up, it causes toxins to be flushed back into the liver, pancreas, and gallbladder. The toxins then re-enter the blood stream, causing serious toxic overload leading to illness and cancer.

Metabolic Belly Fat

The body is quite resourceful in its endeavors to keep us alive. One of the ways it deals with toxic overload is to create fat cells to store toxins. Stop and think about this for a moment – not only do we hate that extra belly fat hanging around our middle, but it isn't *only* fat, it's saturated toxic waste!

AND – not only is belly fat full of toxic waste, it is 'metabolic' in nature, which means it is alive! That's right, it has a mind of its own, and it thinks it is *starving!* Some extremely overweight people experience hunger all the time – because their *FAT* IS *HUNGRY!*

Eating the SAD GMO infused diet, with little to no nutritional value, causes leaky gut and starves the body of nutrition. This creates a vicious cycle of feeling hungry and eating more non-nutritious toxic ridden SAD food. The body creates more hungry fat cells to store toxins, while it continues to be starved for nutrition. Now the body AND metabolic fat are sending hunger signals, so even more SAD food is eaten, perpetuating the downward spiral into obesity and illness. Is it any wonder someone dies every 51 seconds from heart disease??

One of the reasons people experience unpleasant symptoms when they go on a cleansing fast or detox is because the body is ridding itself of copious amounts of toxic waste stored in their fat cells.

Cholesterol is Not the Enemy!

Leaky gut causes inflammation, and the blood becomes sticky with undigested protein particles and toxins in the bloodstream. This weakens the cellular bonds and damages interior walls of blood vessels and arteries. This damage activates the body's defense mechanism to produce cholesterol. Cholesterol is the body's patching substance for blood vessels and arteries.

> **The vilification of cholesterol is less about heart health and more about pharmaceutical company profit. Cholesterol drugs are a $30 BILLION dollar a year business.**

Healing a leaky gut and getting rid of inflammation in the body will naturally reduce cholesterol numbers. Extremely high cholesterol numbers mean there may be a problem with the liver, not the heart. Again, changing to a non-SAD lifestyle is the best way to heal the liver and reduce cholesterol numbers.

Top GMO Foods to Avoid and What You Must Eat Organic

1. **Soy** – 94% of U.S. crops are GMO
2. **Corn** – 88% of U.S. crops are GMO including high-fructose corn syrup and corn sugar. It used to be that GMO corn was only used for animal feed and in processed foods, but in 2012 Monsanto was able to market sweet Bt Round Up Ready corn – This means corn on the cob! Walmart has chosen to sell this corn and is not required to inform their customers it is GMO.
3. **Canola** (Rapeseed) 90% of U.S. crops are GMO
4. **Sugar Beets** (and sugar made from sugar beets instead of cane) 95% of U.S. crops are GMO
5. **Hawaiian Papaya** – 95 % of U.S. crops are GMO
6. **Zucchini** – 11 % of U.S. crops are GMO
7. **Crookneck Squash** – 11% of U.S. crops are GMO
8. **Apples** – recent approval, Golden Delicious – *Arctic Non-Browning* Apples now in grocery stores in the Midwest
9. **Potatoes** – three brands of GMO potatoes; *Russet Burbank, Ranger Russet and Atlantic*, have been approved and will be showing up in the grocery stores by Fall, 2017.
10. **Salmon** – It's taken nearly 20 years but AquaAdvantage salmon will soon be served in restaurants and appearing at your local fish counter. AquaAdvantage is a manmade breed of salmon that's part Atlantic salmon and part Chinook salmon with a few genes from other fish thrown in. These genetic modifications speed up the animal's growth process by keeping them active most of the year as opposed to only part of the year. The manufacturer claims their salmon grow at twice the rate of farm-raised fish.
11. **Tomatoes** – VEGANS BEWARE! Coming soon – GMO tomatoes engineered with pig and salmon genes to prevent bruising and freezing during transport.

New GMO foods currently in production and seeking approval to appear in a grocery store near you:
- Wheat
- Rice
- Bananas

ORGANIC VS. CONVENTIONAL PRODUCE

The Dirty Dozen & Clean Fifteen

Conventionally grown produce contains high levels of pesticides that cannot be rinsed off because the plant has 'ingested' – or absorbed these pesticides in its flesh during the growing process.

It is best to eat organic whenever possible – but if your food budget is already stretched thin, you can follow the Environmental Working Group's (EWG) advice of which products should always be purchased organic, and which products are not quite so bad if you must buy conventionally grown produce.

Every year the EWG publishes a study disclosing the level of pesticides found in produce. They have created a list called the "Dirty Dozen" which are the twelve most highly polluted produce items you really need to buy organic. And the "Clean Fifteen" which is a list of produce that are not quite as bad to buy conventionally grown.

"DIRTY DOZEN" Always Buy Organic	
• Strawberries	• Cherries
• Spinach	• Grapes
• Nectarines	• Celery
• Apples	• Tomatoes
• Peaches	• Sweet bell peppers
• Pears	• Potatoes

"CLEAN FIFTEEN" OK To Buy Conventionally Grown	
• Sweet Corn*	• Asparagus
• Avocados	• Mangos
• Pineapples	• Eggplant
• Cabbage	• Honeydew Melon
• Onions	• Kiwi
• Sweet peas frozen	• Cantaloupe
• Papayas*	• Cauliflower
• Grapefruit	

A small amount of sweet corn, papaya and summer squash sold in the United States is produced from genetically modified seeds. Buy organic varieties of these crops if you want to avoid genetically modified produce.

Arsenic is fed to poultry and hogs to make their flesh an appetizing pink!

FACTORY FARMED ANIMAL FOOD

Factory farming messes with nature in every way. Deliberately feeding poison to animals so their flesh is a more appetizing color reveals the depths of corruption this industry sinks to.

Factory farming is the industrialization of animals for food. *BILLIONS* of animals are slaughtered each year. Cows, chickens, pigs, turkeys and fish are raised in cramped, unsanitary, conditions.

Factory farming is cruel and abusive. If Americans understood the level of depravity and greed exhibited in the animal food industry the outcry of protest and boycotting meat would force reforms to this grisly business.

The few brave souls venturing into factory farms and taking forbidden video footage of the abuse, rampant disease and suffering of these animals is enlightening for those who choose to see.

Factory Farmed Fish

Farmed fish are raised in near shore polluted water and get sea lice and parasites because they are corralled in small spaces and live in their own feces.

Factory farmed fish are given antibiotics and fed GMO corn and soy. This IS NOT a natural diet for fish – when have fish in nature ever eaten an ear of corn? Or a soybean? The farther away we get from nature, the more contaminated and unhealthy our food supply becomes.

The healthy benefits of eating wild caught salmon are lost on farmed fish. Only *wild* salmon is rich in Omega-3 fatty acids because wild salmon eat algae rich in Omega-3's.

So be sure that all fish you eat is wild caught.

Remember, unless otherwise stated, all beef, pork, chicken, eggs, dairy and fish you eat at restaurants and fast food establishments are factory farmed and loaded with preservatives, pesticides, toxins, hormones and antibiotics.

ANTIBIOTICS AND HORMONES

Poultry

According to the U.S. Department of Agriculture, the poultry industry raises nearly 9 billion broiler chickens and 80 million turkeys each year. 90% of all antibiotics produced in the U.S. are used on animals because of diseases rampant in industrial farm conditions.

Hormones, antibiotics and caffeine are added to the food and water of poultry. This increases their breast size, helps them survive their filthy living conditions and stay awake to eat constantly and grow to market size faster. The skin of these chickens is loaded with anti-microbial resistant bacteria combatting the load of ingested antibiotics.

Prozac, an anti-depressant drug, is given to chickens to calm them down in the intense overcrowding conditions.

> **Studies show that poultry workers slaughtering and handling dead chickens are 9 times more likely to develop hormone related cervix, penis, and pancreatic cancer.**

The effects on the human body when ingesting animals treated with antibiotics and hormones accumulate over time. These effects will show up in your body – it is just a matter of when, depending on the strength of your digestive system and how sensitive you are to chemicals, antibiotics and hormones.

The negative effects on our bodies from eating contaminated chicken are intensified when chicken is coated with GMO breading and deep frying in GMO oil. Eating deep fried skin on chicken LOADED with millions of microbiome fighting bacteria greatly increases your chances of developing debilitating disease. Fried chicken fast food is not the best option for you and your families' health.

Dairy Cows – GMO Milk *Doesn't* Do a Body Good!

Hormones are given to milk cows to force their overworked bodies to create more milk. Some hormones that are used in dairy cows include:

- Recombinant bovine growth hormone (rBGH) A Monsanto developed GMO – or bovine somatotropin (BST) is used to promote milk production.
- Estrogen, testosterone, and progesterone – hormones are given to promote growth and production.
- Steroid additivities are also administered to increase growth and development.

The FDA approved rBGH in 1993 despite criticism that the effects of rBGH were never properly assessed. The FDA's approval was based solely on studies administered by Monsanto – rBGH was tested for 90 days on 30 rats. Although the FDA stated the results showed no significant problems, the study was never actually published.

In 1998, an assessment by Health Canada determined that the results of Monsanto's 90 day study provided reason for review before approval of rBGH. Today the EU, Japan, Australia, New Zealand and Canada do not allow the use of rBGH, due to animal and human health concerns. The U.S. is the only western, industrialized nation to allow rBGH.

Certainly there is enough controversy and related test studies claiming links to cancer, obesity, and the onset of early puberty related to rBGH to warrant us removing it from our diet.

Multi-Drug Resistant Bacteria

Bacteria are living micro-organisms that battle our immune system for supremacy in our bodies. The "miracle" of penicillin launched medical science into a new era of discovery. It was believed life-threatening bacteria was now on the run and would soon cease to be a threat to humanity. However, nature has a way of surviving, and if you try to conquer it, it will fight back, with a vengeance.
In the beginning penicillin saved thousands of lives. It was introduced in 1938, but by 1945 resistant strains of bacteria began appearing.

We now know that each new strain of antibiotic introduced to the population quickly generates drug resistant bacteria. '*Ciproflaxacin*' a broad spectrum antibiotic introduced in 1968 developed resistant bacterial strains that same year. *Diarylquinolines*, a narrow spectrum antibiotic introduced in 2006, developed resistant bacterial strains by 2012.

(http://www.nature.com/nrd/journal/v12/n5/fig_tab/nrd3975_T1.html)

Antibiotic resistance means the germs and bacteria we are seeking to kill are becoming immune to the antibiotic drugs we are using to combat them. Therefore more and more antibiotics are given to animals – and to humans – in the fight against disease while bacteria become stronger and stronger in order to survive.

Chapter 7

Sugar – The Sweet Silent Killer

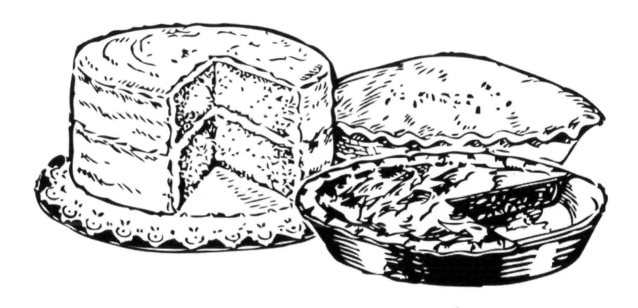

Ah sugar – that sweet, delectable darling we crave, enjoy and overindulge in – and unfortunately, are addicted to. The more we eat, the more we want. And the sicker we become.

For me – when I go through periods of detoxing and eating right, I don't crave sugar. I have lots of energy and feel great. I don't even think about sugar. However, if I open the door to sugary treats on vacation or a weekend with friends, the cravings return. I know I must resist these cravings or old habits will take hold again and lead to the downward spiral of gaining back unwanted pounds and inches.

Sugar feeds cancer, causes degenerative illness, obesity and premature aging. I've heard it said – *sugar makes you fat, sick and stupid!*

Sugars are carbohydrates composed of carbon, hydrogen, and oxygen. Sugars come in a variety of forms that can be distinguished easily under a microscope by their chemical structure. The body recognizes these structures and processes each differently.

GLUCOSE and FRUCTOSE have distinct molecular structures that react very differently in the body. This forces the body to metabolize these two types of sugar and use their energy in very different ways.

GLUCOSE

The MAIN energy source of the body is glucose; it is processed into energy to be used right away or stored as glycogen in the liver and muscles. Glucose is vital for the function of every cell in our body. Glucose comes from the food we eat and beverages we drink.

FRUCTOSE

Fructose is *already* sugar so the body does not need to break it down. Fructose metabolizes instantly into FAT and sends it directly to the belly, hips, breasts and thighs! And – you pay a hefty price of time and energy to get it out!!!

Fructose turning instantly into fat is like the Monopoly board game when you land on the 'go to jail' space. You do not get to collect your $200 – and are penalized to languish in jail until you either roll doubles or pay $50.00 to get out of jail.

This reminds me of a commercial that came out some years ago showing people walking around with bagels and donuts hanging from their under arms, bellies and thighs. This commercial was a perfect example of what happens when we eat the deadly combo of white flour and sugar. This was one commercial I enjoyed, but the manufactures of bagels and donuts were so angry the ad was quickly pulled.

Whole Foods versus Processed Foods

The closer to Mother Nature we eat, the healthier we are. A whole food is a food in its natural state. Grains, nuts, seeds, fruit and vegetables all have fiber, so they take longer to digest and become glucose energy in the body. These foods contain fructose in their natural state, but because they contain fiber, the body processes them into usable energy.

The more a food is processed, the more it has been stripped of its natural goodness of fiber, vitamins and minerals. Highly processed high fructose foods bypass the normal digestive process and quickly become fat.

Highly processed foods have no fiber. Fiber is the substance that helps food move successfully through the intestines and colon for elimination. We want our food passing along at a nice pace, not getting bogged down and staying too long. It's the body's job to extract nutrients from food and eliminate unnecessary waste such as food additives, chemicals and toxins.

When poorly digested food stays in the colon for too long the toxins in the fecal material circulate back through the blood stream into the gallbladder, pancreas, liver and kidneys like a backed up sewer. This overloads vital body organs and, once overloaded, they become diseased, break down and eventually give up.

Think of the damage done to your car if you don't change the oil. The engine filter gets clogged and results in burning up the engine.

Sugar Spikes & Insulin Resistance

When foods containing processed sugar are eaten the body experiences a burst of energy – a high if you will. But what happens soon afterward is the sugar "crash" that leaves you feeling foggy brained, sluggish and wiped out.

* GLUCOSE – Triggers the release of leptin and insulin hormones that signal the brain that you're full.

* INSULIN – Is the hormone that transfers glucose into the cells for utilization. You can think of insulin as the "vehicle" to move the glucose to where it needs to be.

* NATURAL FRUCTOSE – Whole fruits and vegetables contain natural fructose, which is easily utilized in the body as energy.

❖ <u>PROCESSED FRUCTOSE</u> – impacts the body instantly, and *does not* trigger that 'full' signal to the brain, therefore the bingeing of sugar is dangerous and overloads the body with insulin.

Insulin Resistance happens when the body is forced to deal with the excess of insulin production from consuming too much processed sugar, high fructose corn syrup and processed food. The body becomes overloaded with insulin and must 'resist' the effects and benefits of insulin.

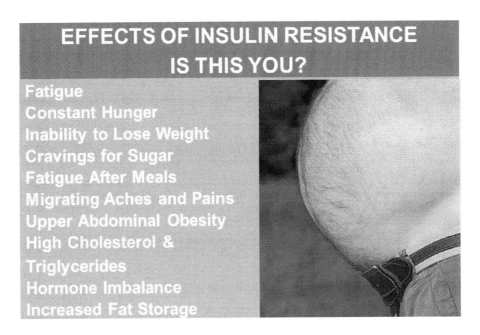

How Much Sugar Are You Eating?

The effects of sugar are cumulative in the body. We talked about sugar spikes – the highs and lows that come from consuming too much processed sugar that you experience soon after eating. But hidden sugars in foods can sneak up on you without even realizing it.

SUGAR MAKES US SICK!		
▪ Increases risk of heart disease	▪ Ages the body	▪ Hair loss
▪ Increases risk of cancer	▪ Hypertension	▪ ADD/ADHD
▪ Increases risk of diabetes	▪ Insomnia	▪ Increases Wrinkles
▪ Tooth decay	▪ Dizziness	▪ #2 Diabetes
▪ Makes us fat	▪ Allergies	▪ Thyroid Disease
▪ Autoimmune Disorders	▪ Heart Disease	▪ Hypoglycemia

The American Heart Association recommends that men eat no more than 36 grams of sugar per day, and women no more than 20.

Sugar Formula:

1 cube of sugar = 1 teaspoon

4 grams of sugar = 1 teaspoon

When reading a food label look at the total sugar grams listed per serving, then divide that amount by 4 to determine how many teaspoons of sugar is in one serving.

For men the daily recommendation is 36 grams – divide 36 by 4 = 9 teaspoons of sugar TOTAL per day.

For women 20 grams divided by 4 = 5 teaspoons.

This is not very much sugar.

Strawberry-flavored original Yoplait yogurt, despite being 99 percent fat free, packs a whopping 26 grams of sugar *per 6-ounce container!!!*

This one little 6 ounce container packs 6.5 teaspoons of sugar – going over the women's daily recommendation by 1.5 teaspoons in a single serving.

Sugar – Is a Highly Addictive Substance

It is being suggested that sugar addiction needs to be addressed and treated as seriously as any other drug addiction. In scientific tests rats preferred the sweet taste of sugar over crack cocaine!

Consuming too much sugar causes eating disorders and changes behavior. Excessive sugar consumption increases dopamine – the happy feel-good chemical in a similar way to opiate drugs. So the sugar "high" feels good for a while, but people desiring to achieve that same high will need to consume higher and higher levels of sugar in order to reach the level of satisfaction they seek. Coming down from a sugar high can cause mild depression, so more sugar is consumed to stop the downward slump into feeling down and unhappy.

Sugar messes with the hormone levels in the body. Going "cold turkey" off sugar will cause discomfort and intense cravings, but if you give the body about three days, it will calm down and begin to produce dopamine normally once again.

Sugar Feeds Cancer

Cancer cells are glucose metabolizers. Being *abnormal cells* with damaged cell biology, they do not absorb nutrition like a normal cell, but require lots of sugar for survival. Cancer cells consume sugar at 10-12 times the rate of healthy cells.

Oncologists are aware of cancer's appetite for sugar and that's why the Positron Emission Tomography (PET) scan uses radioactive glucose to detect cancer cells. When radioactive sugar is injected into a cancer patient – the cancer cells ingest the glucose and light up like a Christmas tree! No lights, no cancer. Intensity of light indicates the severity and location of the cancer.

Rather than telling patients to cut sugar out of their diet because it contributes to the spread of cancer, some oncologists prescribe diabetic drugs to combat high blood sugar. Again, a misplaced Allopathic medical dependence on drug therapy versus simple lifestyle changes to combat disease.

Unfortunately, all drugs come with side effects, and adding even more toxic pharmaceutical drugs to a person fighting cancer – in my opinion – is contributing to illness, not alleviating it.

Body Speak!

Chapter 8

Inflammation – The Fire Within!

Systemic ongoing inflammation in the body is at the root of nearly every disease.

According to Sunil Pai, MD, author of *An Inflammation Nation;*

"The common link among almost every disease and the factor that causes the progression of those diseases is inflammation. From allergies to asthma, from fibromyalgia to arthritis, from colitis to cancer, research now suggest and demonstrates that most, if not all disease begins and worsens with inflammation."

We know we are in big trouble when we feel horrible and develop a fever and body aches and pains. The higher the fever the more virulently our immune system is heating up to battle and overcome the attacking virus or bacteria. Usually fever dissipates within a few hours or a couple days once the immune system has overcome the attack.

Chronic inflammation is the body's perpetual immune system response to exposure to environmental toxins and the effects of eating SAD. This dangerous and prolonged low-grade response is more subtle than a virus attack but shows up in distinct body speak symptoms and chronic disease.

The Immune System

The immune system is the body's first line of defense against disease and foreign substances that come into contact with the body from the outside world. It is the job of the immune system to identify both the good and the bad and activate safety mechanisms to either rid the body of the offending element, or absorb the nutrition and send it along to nourish every cell of the body.

The immune system is an army of cells that defend your body from invaders of every kind of microbe:

- Bacteria
- Viruses
- Yeast
- Parasites
- Spirochetes like Lyme
- Toxins
- Anything that is perceived as 'foreign' – even food

Two-Part Immune System Response

1. The innate immune system: First line of defense and ready to go at all times.

2.   The <u>adaptive immune system</u>: The adaptive system is informed by the innate system to get to work against invaders and it needs time to respond – hours to days – and has memory.

The 'memory' adaptive cells create a permanent 'immunity' for diseases the body has already encountered and conquered. Take chickenpox, for example. When the body overcomes chickenpox, it creates 'soldier cell' antigens that guard the body at all times from the chickenpox virus, the instant these antigens identify the virus they immediately destroy it.

The adaptive immune system is behind the idea of vaccinations and flu shots. These shots are given in the hope the body will create 'memory' soldier cells to combat the diseases the vaccines are designed to fight against.

Immunization vs. Vaccination

In the early days of immunological study, when one person had contracted and overcome a contagious disease, their blood was referred to as the "blood of the overcomer." This blood was considered to be especially rich in antibodies against the infecting agent of the disease. It was used to create 'convalescent serum' and made into immunization shots that were quite affective against Smallpox.

The world's first immunization campaign was the Spanish Smallpox Vaccine Expedition of 1803-1813. The smallpox virus 'convalescent serum' was kept alive in orphaned children as they sailed the seas on the king's command to take immunization to his colonies in danger of being wiped out by the disease. The children were infected by the injection of the live virus in small amounts and the convalescent serum was literally transferred from one child's arm to another;

https://www.ncbi.nlm.nih.gov/pubmed/19329842

Immunology using 'convalescent serum' was used to save millions of lives from smallpox, cowpox, and measles in the early days of vaccination.

Immunization, done correctly with substances proven to be safe for humans, saves lives. Modern-day vaccines are loaded with poison and toxins that cause the body to become inflamed and in desperate need of detox. Unfortunately, today's big pharma vaccines and flu shots are not tested before being used on humans and have been shown to cause long-term and irreversible damage. Today's vaccines of toxic soup – some with live virus – and some with dead viruses, contain additives and preservatives including *mercury, MSG* and *aluminum*. These ingredients have been shown to cause autoimmune disease and brain damage – *but that's a topic for another book!*

> **Chronic inflammation happens when the body is in constant vigilance and high alert combating the toxins coming at it from all sides – GMOs, pesticides, pharmaceutical drugs, sugar, fat, salt, artificial food additives, the chemicals in cosmetics, and environmental toxins.**

THE INFLAMMATORY RESPONSE

Inflammation is the natural healing response the body triggers every time it experiences an injury or locates a toxic invader of unknown origin. Our skin is the first barrier of defense for the body. The outside world enters the body through the skin and the mouth. When the skin is cut, the body triggers an inflammatory response by changing blood flow and sending blood, proteins and white blood cells already on patrol in the body to the site of injury. The white cells study the invader and take back the 'image' of the invading microbe to the nearest lymph node and a concoction of disease fighting antibodies are created inside the lymph node to attack and overcome the harmful invaders. This is why the lymph nodes in our neck swell when we become sick. This is a defense mechanism to protect the body from infection. Its purpose is to localize and eliminate the offending agent and remove damaged tissue so the body can begin to heal.

Chronic Inflammation – The Link to All Disease

Once the immune system activates, it does its job to kill microbes and heal the body. It does not back down until the mission is accomplished. When we first become sick – we are miserable and symptoms compile until our body figures it out and kills the invader. Depending on the illness this can take 24 hours to several weeks. But once the offending microbes are conquered all the symptoms subside and life gets back to normal.

Systemic, ongoing inflammation in the body is at the root of nearly every disease. According to Sunil Pai, MD, author of *An Inflammation Nation;*

> *"Regardless of where they are localized in the body and the names that we have given them, all diseases lead back to inflammation. All fields of health science – cellular biology, physiology, biochemistry, and immunology – have been pointing to inflammation as the common link to disease for over a decade."*
>
> *"However, inflammation is not always the cause of disease; it is always the trigger mechanism that makes every health condition worse."*

If you want to live a long and healthy life, you must keep your inflammation as low as possible. Not only does inflammation wreak havoc in the body it accelerates aging!

Important Sources of Chronic Inflammation in the Body:

1. **Food Factors**: sugar, animal proteins – including dairy, grilled or fried foods. The National Cancer Institute studies show cooking meat at high temperatures releases chemicals that increase the risk of cancer.
2. **Environmental Pollutants/Toxic Agents**: black mold, industrial pollutants, fuels, smog, heavy metals, chemotherapy.
3. **Pharmaceutical & over the counter drugs**: taking prescription and over the counter drugs like NSAIDS *(anti-inflammation drugs; aspirin, Celebrex, ibuprofen, alieve, naproxen)* for long periods of time increases the toxic load

in the body and increases inflammation. Also taking NSAIDS on an empty stomach over time can cause ulcers and stomach bleeding.

4. Bacteria
5. Parasites
6. Viruses
7. Tobacco
8. Alcohol
9. Stress
10. Ultraviolet Radiation: the sun, tanning booths
11. Environmental Allergens: grasses, weeds, molds, animals, dust mites

> **Uncontrolled inflammation caused by toxic environmental exposure, poor diet and lifestyle choices, and high levels of stress all affect the onset of chronic diseases, even cancer.**

It is vital to locate all sources of inflammation causing elements in your life. Learning how to put out the fire of inflammation will enable you to enjoy a long, healthy life of vitality and wellbeing.

Inflammation: Food Allergies & Sensitivities

Since 80% of our immune system resides in the gastro-intestinal track (the gut), it is important to understand that certain foods cause inflammation in everyone, and other foods cause specific reactions that are unique to each individual.

Food allergies and sensitivities are a major source of hidden chronic inflammation. Unknowingly, people are eating foods that are causing a war of inflammation in the gut, which spreads out from there to affect every cell in their body.

This is why it is so important to listen – and respond to – our Body Speak.

Allergy vs. Sensitivity

If you are actually allergic to a particular food – you will need to remove that food permanently from your diet.

Food "sensitivity" on the other hand is something you can overcome by removing that food for a period of time. With proper nutrition and long-term monitoring of symptoms, previously offending foods can be re-introduced back into the diet and enjoyed once the leaky gut is healed. See *Fermented Foods That Heal* and the *Elimination Detox Diet* Chapters for ways you can actively support and heal your GI track.

Healthy Gut vs. Leaky Gut

Every food has a unique biological marker – or an ID tag if you will. All food has protein, an amino acid sequence recognized by the immune cells. These cells know the difference between the cells of the human body and the cells of other substances entering the body.

In a healthy gut, food is digested in the stomach by enzymes and acid. All the ID tags that make food recognizable are broken down and rendered unrecognizable from the food ID it once had. This is specifically designed to stop food allergies and sensitivities. The body is not designed to attack itself, or the food it eats.

Here's how it is supposed to work – when a whole-wheat tuna salad sandwich is eaten, the brain and taste buds know what it is, but the stomach does not. The stomach douses the ground up sandwich remains with digestive enzymes and acid, breaking down all the recognizable ID traits of the 'protein amino acid sequence' of the whole-wheat and tuna it just ingested. The body does not say – *Oh hey this is wheat, this is tuna, this is mayo*. The stomach just takes everything it gets and breaks it down into usable nutrients that now hold no recognizable food 'ID tags' to alert the immune system. This is meant to keep the body free from identifying food as an invader. Unless, of course, if food is tainted with salmonella, E.coli, or other harmful bacteria; the body launches full scale war against these deadly invaders – and the content of the stomach is usually discharged violently!

Food is good. Food is necessary to keep us alive. Food is not supposed to create unpleasant reactions in the body. And when the body is healthy and the food is real, whole and natural, food of all kinds can be enjoyed with no adverse reactions.

Problem: Weak Intestinal Lining

When we cut outer skin, an immune response is instantly triggered to heal the source of the tear. It is the same with the inner "skin" lining of the gut. Once there is even an infinitesimal tear in the lining of the gut wall, toxins and undigested food particles leak into the blood stream. Now this unfortunate condition alerts the warrior immune cells, and big trouble begins to occur.

Leaky Gut Syndrome

As previously discussed GMO's and the herbicide glyphosate in Round Up Ready crops have caused an epidemic of leaky gut in our nation. The crops themselves are engineered to live even when saturated with poison. And not only this, the crops ARE ENGINEERED to actually BE THE PESTICIDE that bursts open the guts of the insects that eat them.

When we eat a diet of gut-bursting pesticides, the villi – the tiny 'hairs' in the lining of the entire GI track, become damaged. This causes the cells inside the GI track to become 'permeable' which means they leak and are no longer capable of keeping food particles safely inside the intestines.

Once identifiable food particles enter the blood stream – along with glyphosate and other chemicals and food additives – the immune system identifies these food's ID tags and assigns them as foreign invaders that must be attacked and destroyed.

Indigestion, bloating, gas, irritable bowl, constipation, foggy brain, low energy, acne, sneezing, runny nose and joint aches and pains are all signs of leaky gut, food sensitivities and poor digestive issues.

- Part Three -

HOW

To Recover From

SAD -

Detox & Thrive!

Body Speak!

Chapter 9
The Anti-Inflammatory Lifestyle

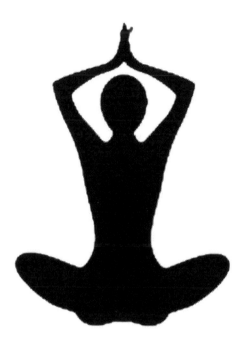

We've discussed how inflammation is like heat – fire, in the body. The goal is to calm the body down and stop the inflammatory response to foods. One of the ways to do this is to understand which foods turn on the 'heat' and which foods 'neutralize' the heat and cool the body down.

Acid & Alkaline Forming Foods

Everything we eat and drink performs a function in our body. Balance is the key to recovering and maintaining health. In Chinese Medicine this is called Qi, the balance of yin and yang.

Different foods create either an 'alkaline' or 'acid' response in the body. Some foods are more 'hot' or acid forming, while other foods are more 'cool' and alkaline forming.

Foods are classified either acidic or alkaline by the mineral content left behind from the metabolic process of digestion. Acidic foods are defined as foods that increase acid waste products in the blood. Alkaline foods are foods that produce ash that neutralizes acid products in the blood.

Acid forming foods increase joint pain and contribute to chronic inflammation which is at the root of all disease, especially cancer.

Consuming an imbalance of acid forming foods throws the pH of the body into turmoil. Acid levels in the body rise due to overconsumption of animal proteins, dairy products, processed foods and sugars. The lungs and kidneys will compensate for above normal acid levels – the body works hard to maintain a pH balance. You can help your body out by understanding how to maintain a balance between acid forming food and alkaline forming food.

A good way to understand what foods form high acid levels is to understand the more protein a food contains, the higher the acid level it produces. When you choose to eat acidic animal foods such as meat, chicken or fish, it is good to design your sides around fresh non-starchy alkaline vegetables and salads.

Quinoa is a high protein grain – but surprisingly – it is alkalizing. Combining meat with a side dish like quinoa loaded with vegetables is a great way to bring acid and alkaline balance to a meal.

Fresh, raw, whole fruits and vegetables are best for alkalizing the body. Any process such as cooking, freezing, canning or preserving with sugars and chemicals greatly reduces the alkaline/acid values of fruits and vegetables. This includes all jams, jellies, and other processed fruit products.

The more processed a food is, the more acid it forms in the body. Whole wheat and brown rice are less acid forming than bleached white flour breads and pastas. The more 'white' a food is the less nourishing it becomes and the more acid it produces in the body.

GRAINS, SEEDS, NUTS: Acid-forming grains, seeds and nuts become alkaline forming when sprouted. There are some naturally alkalizing grains; see table below.

High Acid Forming	Moderate Acid Forming	High Alkaline Forming
All Animal Foods All Dairy	A few vegetables and some grains are higher in acid than others. They are listed below.	Fresh Fruit The sweeter the fruit, the higher the alkaline benefits.
Artificial Sweeteners	Beans – soaked & sprouted	Citrus Fruits; grapefruit
High Fructose Corn Syrup	Grains – soaked & sprouted	lemons, limes, oranges
Barley	Nuts – soaked & sprouted	Dates, fresh & dried
Buckwheat	Pumpkin	Figs, fresh & dried
Corn Meal	Sunflower	Carob Powder
Oats, steel cut	Wheat Germ	Raw Honey
Rice		Agar – a sea vegetable
Rye		Almonds
Spelt		Avocado
Wheat		Garlic – exceptional food!
Liquor		Amaranth
Beer		Millet
Wine		Quinoa
Caffeine Drinks		Herbal tea from leaves
Coffee		All leafy greens
Soft drinks		Sesame, un-sprouted

Alkalizing Herbs: Agave, basil, celery seed, chives, cilantro, dill leaves, marjoram, oregano, rosemary, sage, stevia, tarragon and thyme.

Juicing vs. Blending

Drinking the juice from fresh fruit & vegetables is a great way to alkalize the body and packs a whole lot of nutrition into one serving. Fresh juice is a 'living food' abounding with vitamins, minerals, antioxidants and enzymes.

Whether you blend or juice is up to your personal preference. You can blend in a high power blender and then, depending on what you blend, strain out the fibrous pulp. Or, you can purchase a juicer to separate juice from pulp in one step.

If you do not already have a juicer – check out the Juicer Fanatics website for a list of the top rated juicers. http://www.juicerfanatics.com.

We use an Omega J8006 - because it is a more 'gentle' juicer. It rotates the produce in a moving spiral that extracts the most juice from your valuable produce.

The BEST Juicer is the One You Will Use Daily!

Depending on what you juice, it can be incredibly nutritious and delicious or, nutritious and maybe not so delicious. The juice we drink is the later, for the most part. When Mike was recovering, we developed what we call the "Health Blast" juice, it packs a whole lot of vitamins and nutrients, but it is not a tasty juice. Here is the recipe.

<u>HEALTH BLAST JUICE</u> – *Makes approx. 28 oz.*

- 1/2 red beet
- 3 stalks kale
- 3 celery stalks
- 1/4 bunch cilantro
- 1/4 bunch parsley
- 2 green apples

- 1 lemon - peeled
- 1 orange - peeled
- 3 inches ginger root
- 3 inches turmeric root
- 1/4 jalapeno - seeded

L'chiam! - To Life!

Anti-Inflammatory Supplements & Diet

Helpful supplements include: Vitamin D3, Vitamin A, Vitamin E, Zinc, essential fatty acids; antioxidants, Co-enzyme Q10, Molecularly distilled fish oil.

Essential Fatty Acids (EFAs) are beneficial fats because your body cannot produce them on its own so they must come from your diet. The two primary EFAs are known as linoleic acid (omega-6) and alpha-linolenic acid (omega-3).

Sources of Omega 3's include flax seeds, pumpkin seeds, walnuts and dark green veggies, such as kale, collards, chard, parsley, and cereal grasses (wheat & barley grasses). Green (chlorophyll-rich) foods contain Omega-3 EFA in their chloroplasts.

Sources of Omega-6 fatty acids include nuts, seeds, grains and legumes.

A vegetarian diet is naturally low in fat, so be sure to include EFA-rich foods in your healthy lifestyle.

Source: https://www.downtoearth.org/health/nutrition/benefits-essential-fatty-acids

Healthy Fats:
- Avocado
- Olive Oil
- Coconut Oil
- Ghee

Healthy dietary fat supports every cell membrane in your body and influences function. It is vital for communication between cells and crucial to the immune system. Fatty acids work directly with soldier lymphocyte T cells which are processed by the thymus gland to regulate cell function, immunity and inflammation.

Antioxidants protect the body from damage caused by harmful molecules called free radicals. Many experts believe free radical damage is a factor in the development of blood vessel disease (atherosclerosis), cancer, and other conditions.

Antioxidants are necessary for the following processes:

- Formation of healthy cell membranes
- Proper development and functioning of the brain and nervous system
- Proper thyroid and adrenal activity
- Hormone production
- Regulation of blood pressure, liver function, immune and inflammatory responses
- Regulation of blood clotting: Omega-6 EFAs encourage blood clot formation, whereas Omega-3 oil reduces clotting. The ideal is to achieve a balance between omega-6 and omega-3 EFAs
- Crucial for the transport and breakdown of cholesterol
- Support healthy skin and hair

Foods Rich in Antioxidants:

- Berries
- Cantaloupe
- Grapefruit
- Honeydew
- Kiwi
- Mangoes
- Nectarines
- Oranges
- Papaya
- Strawberries
- Broccoli
- Brussel sprouts
- Cauliflower
- Kale
- Red, green, yellow peppers
- Snow peas
- Sweet potato
- Tomatoes
- Carrots
- Chard
- Mustard greens
- Turnip greens
- Pumpkin
- Spinach
- Nuts
- Sunflower seeds
- Garlic
- Onions

Chapter 10

The Basics of the Modern Healthy Diet & Lifestyle

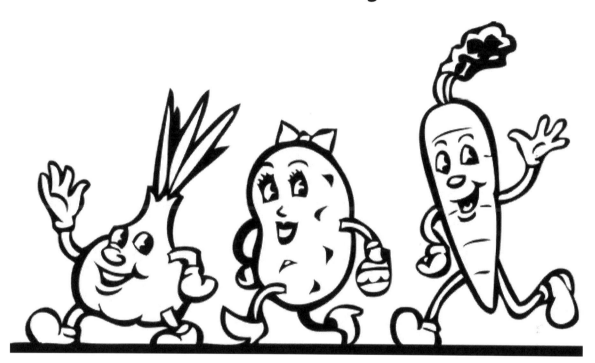

People everywhere want to know…
"What Diet is the *BEST?*"

The fickle waves of diet popularity ebb and flow based upon the latest Amazon and New York Times Best Seller lists. The vacillating masses, all hungering for that elusive formula promising weight loss and a fabulous body, flock to buy whatever is trending at the top of the charts.

If the latest formula offers only a few simple steps to body nirvana or points to eliminating that one villainous food group that is blocking your success – well then people are in and these books fly off the shelves.

Here's the deal, this new 'thing' *will* work for *some* people. Every diet – no matter how crazy – will cause people to release a certain amount of weight. Depending on how crazy or balanced the diet is will determine the sustainability of weight loss. The people who enjoy some success with the latest and greatest formula naturally try to convince others it will work for them too, and the cycle continues.

What do you think? Is there one diet that works for everyone?

At the Institute of Integrated Nutrition (IIN) we learned there is no one diet that is right for everyone. Joshua Rosenthal, Founder, Director and Primary Teacher of IIN uses the term; 'Bio-Individuality' to describe each person's unique needs.

There are basics of nutrition that create optimal health, but the specific way to go about achieving maximum health varies from individual to individual. One person's food is another person's poison.

How do you discover what is best for you? To understand what is healthy and sustainable, one needs to do a little personal *experimentation* and *research*. The Elimination Detox Diet (EDD) provides a process for you to experiment and discover what foods your body can and cannot handle and sustain as a new lifestyle. As to research, find reliable sources who have a long history of healing people and point to nutritional truth, rather than the hyper sensationalism of marketing trends and food industry disinformation. This book is the culmination of my research, and there are many sources of additional information listed at the end of the book.

A Calorie is a Calorie – Or is it?

When I first learned about calories – as a teenager wanting to lose weight – I did not understand that not all calories are equal. I figured if 1 ½ ounces of red vine licorice was 140 calories – with no fat – and an egg on a dry piece of whole wheat toast was about 133 calories, *plus* an egg includes 5 grams of fat, I might opt for the licorice. I would just keep track of all of the calories I consumed in a day and try to stop at 1,000. That was a crazy way to live, but I was a crazy teenager. Early in life I became a habitual dieter always gaining back the weight once the out-of-balance way of eating stopped. I discovered early on diets do not work, because diets are not a sustainable way to live a healthy, happy life.

What exactly is a calorie? And do different types of calories affect our body differently?

In the simplest form – a calorie is a unit of energy. You've probably heard the term "energy in – energy out." People think if they indulge themselves at a meal and work twice as hard at the gym the next day, it will make up for the indulgence. But will it?

It may make up for one or two indulgences, but thinking that you can eat whatever you want and just work it off at the gym is a fallacy. I've watched people over the span of months working hard at the gym, on the elliptical machine for 45 minutes three times a week, plus doing a weight routine and they do not lose weight, or change the shape of their body.

Just ask any athlete working hard to perform their sport at peak physical precision if they believe they can eat whatever they want and just work harder to compensate. It doesn't work like this.

The body is a magnificent bio-machine and it needs what it needs, period. It will do whatever it takes to keep you alive as long as it can, but it has specific requirements to function well. I like to think of my body kind of like a faithful, beloved dog. It loves me and wants to serve me well. It is faithful to care for me. So, I am faithful to care for it.

Calories are units of energy that fuel the body, but not all calories are equal. Some empty sugar, fat and sodium filled calories damage the body and cause inflammation and even cancer. We've already talked about food values and sugar, but I do not suggest you begin counting calories. I suggest you choose foods that are in their most natural forms. When you eat whole foods, you do not need to be too concerned about calories. Your body will naturally balance itself to the weight it wants to be when you feed it good, organic, natural, whole foods.

Another thing that will happen is your taste buds will change when you cut junk food out of your life. You will begin to taste the 'nasty' additives in chips and crackers. When you switch from unhealthy fats to healthy fats, you will begin to taste rancid oil in restaurant food and discern it in processed foods as well. Your body will begin to crave what is good for it, and reward you with more energy and vitality. I ate a BBQ Pringle chip the other day in memory of those days I enjoyed Pringles, I had to spit it out! It tasted like a combination of cardboard and metal. The fake BBQ chemical flavoring left a pasty deposit on my tongue.

Optimal Health & Longevity – The Blue Zones

National Geographic conducted a world-wide study of the longest living communities on the planet. They hired Dan Buettner, a National Geographic Fellow and multiple New York Times bestselling author, to interview the communities with the largest number of people living to be 100 years and older.

Buettner discovered the five places in the world – where people live the longest, and are the healthiest. These communities have been dubbed **Blue Zones**:

1) **Loma Linda**, California – Seventh Day Adventist Community; no meat; active lifestyle of seniors, strong spiritual faith and practice

2) **Nicoya Peninsula**, Costa Rica – Mediterranean Diet

3) **Sardinia**, Italy – Mediterranean Diet

4) **Ikaria**, Greece – Mediterranean Diet

5) **Okinawa**, Japan – Mediterranean Diet

Here is what Buettner has to say after traveling the globe and interviewing centenarians – people over 100 years old, who retain their full mental capacities and enjoy life and their love ones to the fullest:

> *"The calculus of aging offers us two options: We can live a shorter life with more years of disability, or we can live the longest possible life with the fewest bad years. As my centenarian friends showed me, the choice is largely up to us." – Dan Buettner*

Buettner and his team discovered there are common characteristics within these five communities of the longest living, healthiest people:

- Diet & active lifestyle
- Loving, multi-generational family relationships
- Strong community support
- Maintain a spiritual practice

Loma Linda, California: Its members are **Seventh-day Adventists** who shun smoking, drinking, caffeine, dancing and avoid TV, movies and other media distractions.

They also follow a 'biblical' diet focused on grains, fruits, nuts and vegetables, and drink only water. *(Some of them eat small amounts of meat and fish.)* Sugar is taboo, too.

Gary Fraser, a cardiologist and epidemiologist at Loma Linda University and an Adventist himself, has found in studies that Adventists who follow the religion's teachings lived about 10 years longer than people who didn't. It was also found that Pesco-vegetarians in the community, who eat a plant-based diet with up to one serving of fish a day, lived longer than vegan Adventists.

Their top foods include avocados, salmon, nuts, beans, oatmeal, and whole wheat bread.

The other Blue Zone communities eat mostly the Mediterranean Diet.

The Mediterranean Diet

• **Fruits**	• **Nuts**
• **Vegetables**	• **Healthy Fats; Olive Oil**
• **Whole Grains**	• **Fish, Seafood, Sea Vegetables**
• **Beans**	• **Some Lamb**

Oh, and Buettner shared his Mediterranean centenarian friends also enjoy a glass of organic red wine in the evenings!

Here is how Dan Buettner describes the **Blue Zone Diet**:

• **95/5 Rule Eat Plants**	• **Slash Sugar**
• **Limit Meat**	• **Snack on Nuts**
• **Fish is Fine**	• **Sour on Bread***
• **Diminish Dairy**	• **Go Wholly Whole**
• **Daily Dose of Beans**	• **Drink Mostly Water**

> * 'Sour' on Bread means, eat only 100% whole grain breads or authentic sourdough bread made from live cultures. Limit bread to two slices daily. Choose whole grain corn tortillas over flour tortillas. Avoid white flour breads & wraps.

Exercise & Active Lifestyle

Centenarians enjoy a lifestyle that promotes daily physical activity. Walking, bike riding, gym classes and other forms of organized exercise have been shown to increase life expectancy by 4.5 years.

Love & Social Connections

In Okinawa Japan, they form *moais*, or groups of lifelong alliances. When children are five-years-old they are assigned a group of friends in their community who are meant to be intimately involved in their lives – for *all* of their life! These groups provide them with security, financial and emotional support as well as a sense of belonging.

Loneliness is as bad as smoking!!!

Joining with others who support healthy lifestyle behaviors increases the likelihood that you will adopt these positive habits as well.

The Grandmother Affect Studies show that children living with or near grandparents have longer lives and less disease and mortality!

This is one of my favorite statistics because as of today, I have four grandchildren who I am crazy in love with – and spend as much time with as possible. It is our goal to make our home one of the fun-nest, safest, comforting and memorable places in our grandkids lives.

Dan Buettner asked a 103 year old Japanese woman how it feels to hold her great, great, great, granddaughter, over a century younger than herself and she answered, *"It feels like leaping into heaven."*

Body Speak!

Chapter 11
The Protein Controversy

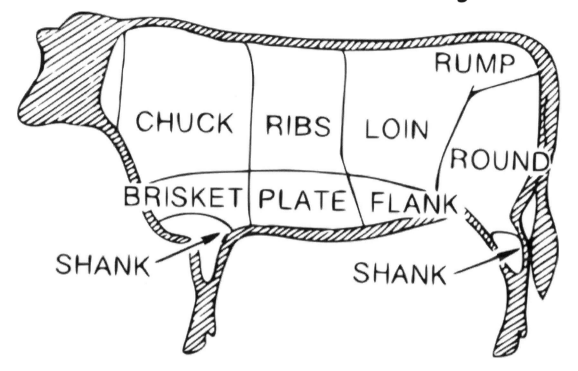

HOW MUCH DO WE NEED – AND WHAT IS THE BEST SOURCE?

One of the first things we heard from our friends and family when we told them we decided to go vegan was, *"But what about protein?"*

We have all heard about the importance of eating enough protein in our daily diet. But how much protein do we really need? And, what protein source is best for the human body?

Many nutritionists agree there's exaggerated hype and worry over the perceived lack of protein in people's diets. The reality is, if you consume enough calories, you're probably eating plenty of protein. The answer lies in what our individual body needs. Not every *'body'* is the same, and there is no one diet that is 'right' for everyone.

"WHERE'S THE BEEF?"

In January, 1984 Wendy's launched a fun and clever TV commercial featuring character actress, Clara Peller. Three elderly ladies standing at a fast-food counter open a great, big fluffy white hamburger bun to find an itty-bitty, round flat burger patty hidden inside the bun and Clara demands; *"Where's the beef?"*

This catchy slogan and Wendy's signature 'square' hamburger patty was in direct competition against the big boys – McDonald's Big Mac and Burger King's Whopper. Creating a square patty – that stuck out from the bun to 'prove' the luscious quality of the meat, brought a novel 'gimmick' to the burger sales competition.

Now, do square hamburgers taste better? Is there actually any reason to sell square hamburgers? Nope. But it makes for a novel change from the others.

> **Whoever has the most money for TV advertisement influences the top of the trending food charts. The truth is out there! We just need to search to find it, and experiment with our own health until we find the solution for what is best for our own lives.**

Marketing Dollars Influence Trends in Nutrition

It is important to understand how media marketing dollars influence what Americans believe about health, nutrition and diet.

We've discussed the 'Misinformation Wars' – and the 'Food Fight' of advertising dollars. There is so much controversial information out there – enough to make the most conscientious researcher a confused basket case!

Protein – how much and what type is best is a hot topic of debate; mostly because the beef and dairy industry pours copious amounts of money into the advertising market.

PROTEIN - Why Is It Important?

Protein is a component of food and is made up of amino acids. It is crucial for vital functions, regulation, and maintenance of our bodies. Amino acids are the building blocks for major parts of a lean human body. Protein comes in many different forms - both from vegetarian and non-vegetarian sources.

Our body makes its own supply of amino acids and also must get some from food. The term 'complete protein' is used to describe sources of protein that contain sufficient amounts of all the essential amino acids necessary for your dietary needs.

Protein is the basic building block of cells and tissues that are needed to keep us strong.

How Much Protein 'Content' Do We Need?

Protein content is the actual amount of 'usable' protein available in food. It is important to understand the difference between protein and protein content.

The U.S. Department of Agriculture's Recommended Daily Allowance (RDA) of protein content for men and women over the age of 19 is 0.36 grams of protein content per each pound of body weight. This means a 130 pound person needs to consume about 47 grams, or 1.7 ounces of actual protein content per day.

Just because you eat a 3.5 oz. hamburger patty, does not mean you are eating 3.5 oz. of protein. For example, a 3.5 oz. hamburger patty contains about 0.58 ounce of protein content, or about 1/3 of the RDA for a 130 lb. person. Actual protein content for a 3.5 ounce portion of various protein sources is shown at the end of this chapter.

Optimal Protein for *Active* Lifestyles

If you are *very active* the RDA can be doubled for 'optimal protein', a concept that more than 40 nutrition scientists promoted at a recent Protein Summit. Their findings were published in 2015 in *The American Journal of Clinical Nutrition.*

An active lifestyle requiring 'optimal protein' means getting at least 35 to 40 minutes of moderate exercise four or five days a week, including resistance training two or more times a week. Research suggests doubling the RDA is best for rebuilding muscle tissue, especially if you do a lot of high-intensity workouts.

Eating more protein as you get older may help you maintain muscle and ward off osteoporosis. According to the above mentioned study, adults over the age of 50 who roughly doubled the RDA (eating 0.68 grams per pound of body weight) were better able to rebuild and retain muscle compared with control groups eating the RDA.

The figure below shows recommended protein and 'optimal' protein content consumption per day in ounces per pound of body weight. Depending on your personal situation, protein content consumption somewhere between the two lines is probably optimal.

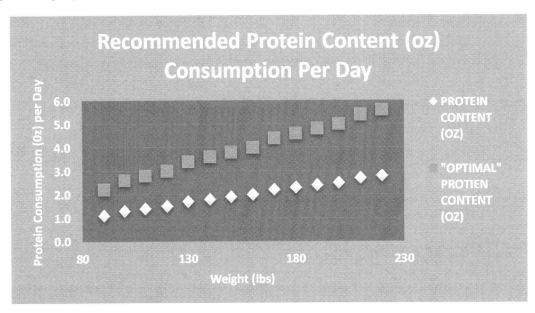

Meat is Not Better Than Plant-Based Protein

Protein is made up of 20 amino acids. Eleven are produced by the bodies of animals and humans, and nine must come from external sources. Meaning animals and humans must get these amino acids from plants since their bodies cannot create them. Therefore, you don't have to eat an animal to get sufficient protein, plants contain all you need. Eating acidic animal food carries the additional burden to your body of digesting toxins and hormones. Even protein from animal food is from plants, so why eat the middle man?

Too Little Protein

Living in America, one is hard pressed *not* to consume sufficient protein – without even trying. The human body needs far less protein than advertisers have led us to believe. Common symptoms of insufficient protein include sugar and sweet cravings, feeling spacey and jittery, fatigue, weight loss, loss of healthy color in facial area, feeling weak, anemia, change in hair color and texture, skin inflammation (*in severe cases*), and potbelly (*in severe cases*).

Too Much Protein

Eating too much protein, say, eating hundreds of grams a day, can lead to trouble according to research. Common symptoms include low energy, constipation, dehydration, lethargy, heavy feeling, weight gain, sweet cravings, feeling 'tight' or stiff joints, foul body odor, halitosis, and calcium loss to compensate for acidic status in body.

HIGH PROTEIN – KETONIC DIETS Can be Dangerous

High protein, low carb diets like Atkins, or high protein Paleo are not as good for your body as the trending hype declares.

As your body digests protein, it produces nitrogen as a by-product, which your kidneys have to process and eliminate as urine. Therefore, large amounts of animal protein can put a strain on your kidneys. And they're not the only organs affected - certain sources of protein can hurt your heart too. A recent Harvard School of Public Health study found that having one small serving of red meat a day increases your chances of dying from cardiovascular disease and other causes by 13 percent, while consuming processed meat, like bacon and hot dogs, ups your chances by 20 percent.

ANIMAL FOOD PROTEINS

It is your choice whether or not to eat animal foods. And, this is a big decision considering today's unsanitary factory farming practices.

**You may be wondering – which is better?
Chicken or Beef?
I just have to share this here – recently while watching the informative documentary; *"What the Health?"* Dr. Caldwell Esselstyn, MD, Cardiovascular Prevention Program, Cleveland Clinic Wellness Institute was asked this question. He answered,**

"Well, depends, do you want to be shot or hung?"

HEALTHY PROTEIN CHOICES

Animal Choices of Protein

Choose Quality: If you choose to consume animal protein, quality is important. The health of the animal affects the health of the consumer. When choosing to eat animal foods it is very important to choose organic, grass-fed beef, organic free-range chickens, raw, organic dairy, and wild caught fish.

It must be said here, the ocean has become quite a polluted environment and wild caught fish are loaded with mercury and other toxins, so be aware of this when eating fish.

Limit Quantity: Generally, animal protein portions should be limited to the size of your palm or smaller.

Digestion: To help digest animal protein, eat plenty of greens and leafy vegetables with your meal. The old adage 'meat & potatoes' is not a good idea. Meals heavy in meat and starch are difficult to digest because meat is highly acidic, and starchy vegetables turn quickly to glucose. These kinds of meals increase inflammation in the body and can lead to constipation and malabsorption.

Energy Type: Many scientific researchers believe a protein is a protein is a protein, whether it is from dry beans, chicken, or a hamburger. But others find that each protein source affects us differently on an energetic level.

As you experiment with various protein sources, pay close attention to see if you notice a difference after eating red meat versus chicken, or wild caught fish. Compare the energy level to when you eat a meal that is solely plant based. You should notice changes in your energy levels depending on the protein source and your specific body needs.

HEALTHY BALANCE OF PROTEIN SOURCES

Low Carb fad diets, such as the popular Paleo and Ketogenic Diets, encourage an increase in protein and fat consumption and a reduction in dairy, carbohydrate and grain intake. In nutrition, balance is necessary to achieve optimal health and wellbeing.

Vegan Sources of Protein

Grains: Whole grains, high in protein and fiber, have been the staple food of civilizations around the world for millennia. Modern refined grains like white flour and white rice have had their bran and germ removed which strips them of naturally occurring vitamins, minerals, and fiber. Whole grains such as brown rice, millet, quinoa, buckwheat, and oats still contain these nutrient-rich components.

Nuts: Nuts are generally considered a heart-healthy fat, not a protein, and are high in fatty acids, fiber, vitamin E, and antioxidants. Peanuts, which are actually legumes, are far higher in protein than most nuts.

Beans: Beans contain a more complete set of amino acids than other plant foods. When first introducing beans into the diet, choose beans that are smaller in size, such as split peas, mung, and adzuki beans, for easier digestion. Digestibility can be further improved by soaking beans overnight, adding spices or vinegar, skimming off the cooking foam, pressure cooking or puréeing, and eating small portions.

> ### *ORGANIC SOY ONLY!!!* Soybeans are one of the most genetically engineered crops, so it is important to choose organic if you choose to eat soy.

Soy: Many vegans and vegetarians use soybeans as a major protein substitute for animal foods. As previously discussed, soy is not considered a healthy food choice by some nutritionists and naturopaths. Soybeans are the most difficult bean to digest. Common forms of soybeans include edamame (baby soybeans), tofu (soybean curd), and fermented soybeans in the forms of tempeh, miso, and tamari.

Fermented is the best way to consume soy for most people unless they have problems with fermented foods. Today's trend to consume soy in various unnatural, highly processed ways like commercial soy milk, soy meat, and soy ice cream may not be a good idea. Many people are allergic to soy.

Soy Milk: Soy milk is highly processed unless it is homemade. If you love the taste of soy milk, drink *organic*.

Non-Dairy Milk: Non-dairy milks such as; coconut, almond, hemp, oat and rice milk are highly processed alternatives to cow's milk. Read ingredient labels and keep these milks to a minimum as some contain preservatives and sugar.

Seitan: Also called 'wheat-meat,' seitan is a high-protein product made from wheat gluten. Seitan is not a whole food, but is not overly-refined either, especially if it's homemade. *(Because this product is pure gluten, it is not a choice for Celiac's or those who are gluten-sensitive).*

Leafy Greens: Broccoli, spinach, kale, collard greens, bok choy, romaine lettuce, and watercress all contain varying amounts of protein. Leafy greens are highly associated with longevity since they contain major sources of magnesium, iron, and calcium. They are a rich source of quercetin, a bioflavonoid with antioxidant, anti-inflammatory, and cancer fighting properties. Green leafy vegetables are dense with easily assimilated amino acids as well as other life-extending nutrients.

Seeds: High in nutrients and lower in caloric content than nuts, seeds provide anti-inflammatory and cardiovascular benefits. Seeds contain vitamin E, fiber, and are some of the few plant-based sources of omega-3s. Some of the healthiest seeds include chia, flax, hemp, pumpkin, sesame, and sunflower.

How can I make sure I am eating the right amount of protein?

The following Table lists sources of protein and how much actual protein content is in a 3.5 ounce (100 gram) serving. After using the figure earlier in the chapter to determine the amount of protein content recommended for you, this Table can help determine the amount of protein content in the particular foods you are eating. Most nutritionists agree that it is best to split protein consumption as evenly as possible between your three daily meals. As you can see, it is not necessary to eat any animal protein to easily meet your body's protein intake needs.

PROTEIN SOURCE	PROTEIN CONTENT (OZ) IN 3.5 OZ SERVING
MEAT	
Beef Top Sirloin	1.07
Bologna (Chicken)	0.36
Chicken Breasts	0.79
Frankfurter (Beef)	0.41
Hamburger Patty	0.58
Lamb Loin Chop	0.71
Turkey Breast	0.52
FISH	
Cod	0.63
Orange Roughy	0.8
Salmon Fillet	0.76
Sardines	0.76
Tilapia	0.85
Tuna Fish (Steak)	0.9
DAIRY	
Cheddar	0.81
Cottage Cheese	0.44
Eggs	0.44
Feta Cheese	0.5
Greek Yogurt	0.35
Mozzarella Cheese	0.86
Parmesan Cheese	1.26
Swiss Cheese	0.95
VEGETABLES	
Bok Choy	1.5
Broccoli	2.8
Collard Greens	3
Green Peas	0.84
Kale	4.3
Romaine Lettuce	1.2
Spinach	2.9
Watercress	2.3

PROTEIN SOURCE	PROTEIN CONTENT (OZ) IN 3.5 OZ SERVING
LEGUMES	
Black Beans	0.76
Chickpeas	0.72
Kidney Beans	0.86
Lentils	0.87
Lima Beans	0.76
Navy Beans	0.79
Soybeans	1.29
Tempeh	0.72
SEEDS	
Chia Seeds	0.58
Flaxseed	0.65
Hempseeds	1.11
Pumpkin Seeds	1.07
Sunflower Seeds	0.73
Tahini	0.6
NUTS	
Almonds	0.74
Cashews	0.64
Peanuts	0.91
Pine Nuts	0.48
Pistachios	0.71
Walnuts	0.54
GRAINS & BREADS	
Buckwheat	0.44
Couscous	0.45
Millet	0.39
Oats	0.48
Quinoa	0.5
Seitan	0.87
Whole Grain Bread	0.47
Whole Wheat Pasta	0.49
Wild Rice	0.52

Chapter 12

Probiotics & Fermented Foods That Heal

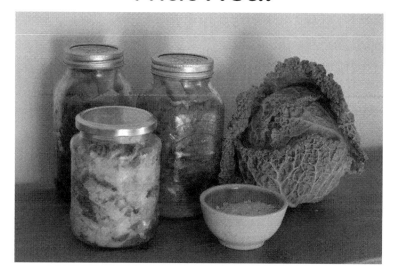

Probiotics are bacteria that line our digestive tract and support the body's ability to absorb nutrients and fight infection. Fermented foods heal and restore the gut and boost the immune system

The outside world enters into the inner sanctum of the body three ways:

1. The skin, the first line of defense and the outer barrier of the body
2. The nose in the air we breathe
3. The mouth in the food and beverages we consume

Our digestive tract is critical to our health because 80 percent of our entire immune system is located in the digestive tract! The gut is home to 100 trillion living bacteria comprised of 400-1000 different species. This microbiome is referred to as the gut flora and works to keep us healthy by supporting digestion and gobbling up the bad bacteria that enter the mouth through food and drink.

The gastrointestinal (GI) tract is the primary site of the interaction between the 'host' immune system – meaning the good bacteria already present in the GI, and the incoming microorganisms from the outside world. When the immune system becomes dysfunctional because of damaged gut flora and leaky gut, many non-infectious human diseases occur such as autoimmunity, allergy, inflammatory bowel disease and cancer.

In addition to the impact of the immune system on gut flora, the digestive system is the second largest part of our *neurological system*. It's called the 'enteric nervous' system and is located in the gut. This is why the gut is called our second brain! Have you ever just 'felt' it in your gut? Or had a friend say when they found out something bad had happened – *"I just felt it in my gut."*

The gut reacts to emotional pain, sorrow, loss and trauma and can cause physical illness. When people experience trauma they lose their appetite and can become severely depressed. Cancer has been linked to high levels of stress, the emotional impact of traumatic loss and the disappointments of life. Just a little 'food' for thought here, pun intended. Keeping the immune system and GI tract strong helps to ride the waves of life's biggest upsets, the kind we can't really prepare for ahead of time. But we CAN work to keep our GI tract strong and healthy in order to support us in whatever life brings our way.

PROBIOTICS

One of the best ways to heal a leaky gut and strengthen the immune system is to go on an Elimination Detox Diet. And, to eat high-quality, colonizing probiotics found in fermented foods.

Probiotic benefits include healing digestive issues, neurological disorders and mental health problems; plus, probiotics boost the immune system and destroy harmful bacteria.

SEVEN REASONS TO EAT FERMENTED FOODS:

1. Heal Digestion
2. Detoxify the Body
3. Increase Energy
4. Boost Immune Health
5. Joint Care
6. Cancer Prevention
7. Weight Loss

Here is a list of the ten top fermented foods that heal and restore the gut and boost the immune system:

Ten Top Fermented Foods:

1. Kefir: A fermented milk drink using grains as a yeast/bacterial fermentation starter. It is prepared by using cow, goat or sheep milk with kefir grains. To make Kefir from non-animal sources such as coconut milk try making your own with Cultures for Health – an awesome company making starter cultures; www.culturesforhealth.com/kefir.

2. Kombucha: A fermented beverage of black tea and sugar from various sources including cane sugar, fruit or honey. It contains colonizing bacteria and yeast that are responsible for initiating the fermentation process. After fermentation, Kombucha becomes slightly carbonated and contains vinegar, b-vitamins, enzymes and a high level of probiotics. Store bought Kombucha can get pricey – check out how to make your own at Cultures for Health; www.culturesforhealth.com/kombucha.

3. Sauerkraut: A crunchy, tangy, probiotic food made from cabbage using a process called lacto-fermentation. Simply put, there are beneficial bacteria present on the surface of cabbage, and in fact, all fruits and vegetables. Lactobacillus is one of those bacteria that once submerged in a brine, begins to convert sugars in the cabbage into lactic acid; this is a natural preservative that inhibits the growth of harmful bacteria.

4. Pickles: Pickling has been used for thousands of years to preserve food beyond the growing season. Pickling cucumbers is most common in the U.S., but in other parts of the world all kinds of fruits and vegetables are pickled.

5. Miso: A fermented 'cake-like' soy used in Miso Soup and other Japanese dishes. The fermentation of soy is vital to break down the daidzein and genistein compounds found in soy that make it difficult to digest.

6. Tempeh: A traditional soy product originating in Indonesia. It is made by a natural culturing controlled fermentation process that binds soybeans into a cake form.

7. Natto: Another form of fermented soybeans — except this process leaves the soybeans intact. Natto creates an enzyme called nattokinase, which produces vitamin K2. Natto is very popular in Japan, but is an acquired taste here in the states — as it has a pungent aroma and the fermented beans are gelatinous in texture.

8. Kimchi: A traditional fermented probiotic food that is a staple Korean side dish. Again, this is an acquired taste for most westerners.

9. Raw Cheese: Raw milk cheeses are made with milk that hasn't been pasteurized. Goat milk, sheep milk and A2 cows soft cheeses are particularly high in probiotics, including thermophillus, bifudus, bulgaricus and acidophilus. If lacto-intolerant, and raw cow's milk cheese is not an option, try goat milk raw cheese to see if you can tolerate and enjoy it.

10. Yogurt: It is important to buy plain yogurt, as flavored fruit yogurts are high in sugar. It is okay to add your own fruit, or to add yogurt to fruit smoothies for added health benefits. Try to buy organic goat or sheep milk yogurt from grass-fed animals. You can also buy or make your own coconut milk yogurt using a starter from Cultures for Health; www.culturesforhealth.com/yogurt. Coconut yogurt is a great substitute for sour cream.

Chapter 13

Detox & Colon Health

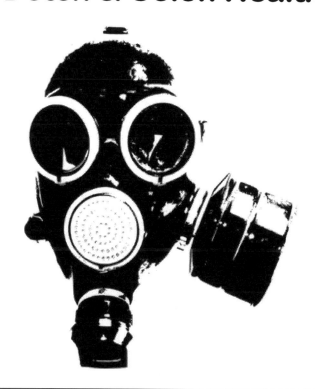

DETOX – is nurturing your body by giving it what it needs to get rid of toxins accumulated through the previous months, years, or even a lifetime.

DETOX IS VACATON FOR THE BODY

When I choose to detox – I am giving my body the vacation it needs to 'clean out the desk.' Our body needs periodic detoxification to heal in the same way we take vacations from work to replenish our psyche.

Detox lessens the body's work load, giving it time to spend its energy on cleaning and repairing vital organs. By eliminating hard to digest foods and adding in whole nutrient rich foods, the body's energy is freed up to flush out accumulated toxins in tissues and cells. Detoxing cleanses the colon and revitalizes the blood, lungs, liver, pancreas and kidneys to work optimally.

Healthy DETOX is Not Hard

Detox has become one of those 'trending' words filling up social media and internet commercials seeking to sell you products. As with any health issue discussed out there in cyberspace – there is confusion and misinformation.

When we hear the word 'DETOX' we envision harsh restrictions, juice only, or 'miracle' pills and powders. A safe, healthy, healing detox does not need to become a harsh or debilitating detox crisis. Detox is healthy and effective when done correctly.

There are supplements that aid in the process of detox, but there is no need to purchase pills or potions. You can successfully detox the body by eliminating certain foods and juicing with fruits and vegetables as shown in the Elimination Detox Diet (EDD). I have listed reliable resources for helpful natural herbs and nutritional supplements in the **Resource List** at the back of this book if you desire to go deeper into detox.

What is DETOX?

Detox is the natural process of cleansing toxins from the body and regenerating cells. Our bodies detox continuously – with every breath and after every meal. The body creates new blood cells to course through the veins and arteries carrying nutrients into cells, while cleaning out the old, dead cells, waste and toxins.

The body naturally detoxes every day, but taking the time out of our busy lives to intentionally detox our body every six months or so will go a long way to keeping the body clean and working properly.

Why DETOX?

As discussed in this entire exposé – our body must process everything we put in it. GMO's, pesticides, chemical additives, etc. are stored in our major organs and fat cells.

On top of that, we are exposed daily to over 80,000 chemicals in our household and personal care products.

Additionally, there are almost 30,000,000 chemicals in the environment, with new ones being released world-wide every year.

There are millions of toxins in our water, food, and the air we breathe which accumulate in our bodies.

This swamp of toxins must be drained periodically to keep us from degenerative disease.

> **Functional medicine doctors see wonderful results in lowering the blood pressure of their patients by taking them through a series of liver and kidney cleanses. It also reduces arterial plaque build-up.**

Clean Body 'Filter' Systems to Lower High Blood Pressure

High blood pressure is a serious Body Speak symptom. It occurs when the heart needs to work harder to pump blood through plaque filled arteries and congested liver and kidneys.

Prevent Fatty Liver Disease

The liver is similar to the oil filter in a car, when it's clogged, it's *fatty* and congested with stones. Just like the 'oil' sensor on your car, high blood pressure is telling you your body is clogged and needs to detox.

Historically, a fatty or 'cirrhotic' liver – or cirrhosis of the liver, was mostly seen in alcoholics. Today, *"Non-Alcoholic Fatty Liver Disease"* is being diagnosed in 12-year-olds! ABC News reported in 2012 that nearly 10% of today's teens have fatty livers.

Fatty Liver Disease is a growing epidemic of obesity due to the SAD western diet saturated in hydrogenated fats, toxins, pesticides, chemicals and microwaved foods.

A CLEAN COLON IS A HEALTHY COLON!

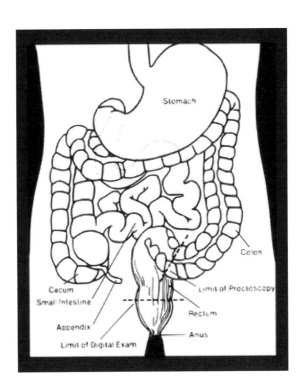

Everything Poops!

Every living thing takes in nutrients to survive, and then poops out the waste. Our cells poop, bacteria poops, and we need to poop – regularly – three times a day or, soon after each meal.

'Clinical' Constipation

If you only poop one time a day – which is probably 2/3 of the population, you are considered to be 'clinically' constipated.

Now, that's something to stop and think about! I thought for years that once a day was okay. And frankly, that once a day did not come out too easily much of the time!

If you only eliminate once a day, this is a DANGEROUS BODY SPEAK SIGNAL!

> **If you are clinically constipated – *do not* ignore or postpone colon intervention. If you go days in between elimination you are in SERIOUS DANGER OF DEVELOPING COLON CANCER! Start a detox program *immediately* to rectify this problem and heal your gut.**

Colorectal Cancer isn't Bad Luck or Genes!

Cancer is preventative – *especially* in the colon! Keep it clean! Keep it running, and it will be smooth sailing for a long healthy life.

Cancer is developed in the colon when old, decayed, rotten food and toxins are not released from the body for long periods of time.

Colorectal cancer is the third most common cancer diagnosed in both men and women in the U.S. The American Cancer Society's estimates for the number of colorectal cancer cases in the U.S. for 2017 are:

- 95,520 new cases of colon cancer

- 39,910 new cases of rectal cancer

Colon cancer is no longer an 'old' people's affliction. I recently heard of a young woman, mom of three young children, in her 30's just diagnosed with stage-four colon cancer. In today's preventative health care model, regular colonoscopies are not suggested until after fifty. And then, these procedures are only repeated every 2 – 4 years. Sadly, many thousands of people clean their colons thoroughly for the first time in their lives *because* they are scheduled for a colonoscopy. And that's after fifty! *Yikes!*

The colon is our body's trash can and should be about 4 inches in diameter, but has the capacity to stretch up to 4 times that size. The wall of the colon naturally 'pulsates' to move fecal matter through. This is called 'peristaltic' motion. Think of it like a healthy muscle able to contract in and out to create motion and move the fecal matter gently through the colon and out of the body.

If food is not digested properly and released out of the colon, the colon stretches and unfortunately – it does not stretch back. When the colon walls are stretched to capacity, they do not 'deflate' back to 4 inches. Plus, the normal peristaltic motion is disrupted because the muscles are stretched too thin to work adequately and move debris out of the body in a timely manner.

Constipation is Dehydration

The body absorbs water and liquid through the colon. If the colon is impacted with old fecal matter, it is difficult to absorb sufficient amounts of liquid into the body. Because of this 'absorption' process in the colon, as the liquid is leached out of fecal matter, that matter becomes more and more hard and difficult to pass down the descending colon and out of the body. It also becomes 'packed' in, and expands, which contributes to painful hemorrhoids and tears with increased effort to eliminate.

90% of the water we absorb into the body is through the COLON. Picture this; a filthy, fecal impacted colon is the *filtering system* you get your water from. Would you ever consider drinking murky brown water polluted with old, toxic fecal matter? I think not. But, this is what happens when we are constipated.

Toxins Recycle Back Through the Blood

Constipation causes toxic fecal matter to pile up in the colon so these toxins recycle through the blood stream over and over again. When toxins are not eliminated and removed from the body through the colon they are stored in our fat cells. The fiber and phytonutrients in fruit and vegetables are naturally detoxifying. When we do not consume sufficient amounts of these detoxifying nutrients, constipation becomes a way of life. Therefore, our blood is dirty and the toxic load continues to build up until the body becomes full of disease and cancer develops.

Irritable Bowel Syndrome – Body Speak Danger Signal!

A healthy bowel movement should be long, narrow, solid, and very easy to pass. And, this should occur shortly after *every* meal. Inconsistent bowel movements going from hard and difficult stools to pass, to urgent spurts of soft stool explosions is considered irritable bowel. This syndrome is indicative of leaky gut and a damaged, distressed digestive system. A damaged digestive system leads to a weak and ineffective immune system and must be detoxified.

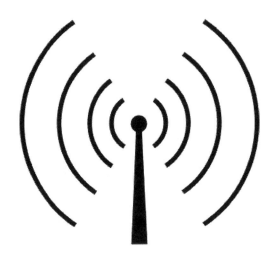

ELECTROMAGNETIC RADIATION – EMR

Everywhere we go, there are 'hidden hazards' of EMR emitted from microwave ovens, cell phones, tablets, TV's, wireless routers, etc. All wireless electronic devices in our homes and ON OUR BODIES *(when we wear our cell phones)* omit invisible energy waves.

EMR energy penetrates the body, just like it penetrates through the walls of our homes, offices, and favorite coffee shops. Modern society's demand for convenience and wireless internet services is putting a toxic burden on our bodies.

Speaking of convenience, microwave ovens cook food with high levels of radiation – which KILLS all nutrients in food. Plus you are exposed to higher levels of EMR while the microwave is operating. We no longer use a microwave and suggest you don't either. Not as convenient, but definitely healthier.

EMR has been associated with a variety of physical and emotional conditions, including multiple sclerosis, ADD, obesity, migraines, anxiety, depression, chronic fatigue syndrome and even cancer.

I share this information with you because of the increasing danger of EMR in the modern age of electronics and wireless technology.

Here is what Ty Bollinger, creator and producer of *The Truth about Cancer*, *The Truth about Vaccines,* and *The Truth about Detox* has to say about EMR:

> *"The 2007 Bio Initiative Report is one of the most important joint reports on EMR and public health. Written by an international group of scientists, researchers, and public health policy professionals, this comprehensive report concluded that there is strong evidence the EMR affects gene expression, induces stress, affects neurological behavior, causes childhood cancers, impacts melatonin production, and reduces immune function.*
>
> *"EMR may be invisible but the associated risks linked to electromagnetic radiation can become all too real with excessive exposure from electronic equipment and wireless networks."*
>
> *Ty Bollinger, The Truth about Detox - https://www.thetruthaboutdetox.com*

Ty goes on to describe what he does in his own home. He utilizes WaveRider technology to create a safe environment for his family. Ty has purchased two WaveRiders, one for each floor of his home. You can check it out here to see if you want to purchase this for your own home http://hado.com/ihm/product/waverider

William Lee Cowden, MD, a USA Board-certified cardiologist, with over twenty years of experience in treating cardiac disease, cancer and other chronic disease, primarily with alternative/integrative medicine, has found invisible electromagnetic frequency to cause cancer in his patients.

At the Truth About Cancer's *Ultimate Live Symposium,* Dr. Cowen shared how a 40-year-old happily married couple presented in his office for a normal evaluation and checkup. Dr. Cowden didn't like what he saw in their blood, so he ordered some more tests that confirmed his suspicions that the husband had colon cancer, and the wife had lymphoma. These people were living a happy life and had *NO SYMPTOMS*. The cancer that had formed in both of their bodies was not from what they were eating, but from what they were being exposed to in their home.

Dr. Cowden sent over a Building Biologist – a technician certified to measure electromagnetic energy in buildings (http://hbelc.org/). The technician discovered 100 times the level approved by the government, and 200 times the level of his own recommendation coursing through the couple's bedroom. The signals were being emitted by two radio alarm clocks at the bedside and a TV. When the tech unplugged these devices, the levels dropped to nearly normal. Dr. Cowden instructed the couple to keep those appliances unplugged for three months. They did what he suggested, came back in after three months for testing – and both were free of cancer! They remained free of cancer for the years Dr. Cowden kept track of them.

Dr. Cowden also suggests not using a metal bedframe, or have any metal in your bedroom. Create a sanctuary of safety when you sleep.

Microwave absorption in our brain from cell phones is greater in children causing necrosis and inflammation. The effects are adaptive and cumulative. Do not hold your cell phone to your ear when you talk. Turn it to speaker and hold it away from your head, or use wired ear buds.

It is important to become proactive in this world of constant EMR exposure. Do not keep your cell phone on next to your bed at night. If you need to have it near you then turn it on airplane mode and set it a distance away from your body. Unplug electronic devices in your bedroom when you go to sleep.

I have included this EMR section to the Detox chapter to inform you of the danger of the constant and accumulative toxic burden of EMR which is in *addition* to all the other reasons for detoxing discussed here.

Chapter 14
HOW TO DETOX

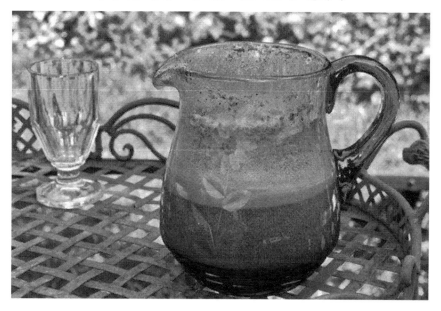

> **There are many levels and ways to go about detoxing the body; everything from adding a few simple things to your daily routine to more advanced intermittent fasting with juice and water.**

Going on the Elimination Detox Diet (EDD) and adding the detox protocols discussed in this chapter will go a long way toward removing toxins from the body. How far you go into detox depends on your personal situation. If you are just beginning to change your lifestyle from SAD to a healthier diet, you need to go slow and easy.

Following these detox protocols during the EDD will release toxins, help you lose weight, strengthen your immune system, calm inflammation and cleanse your colon and blood.

Detoxing From Chemotherapy Drugs and Radiation

If you have already undergone chemotherapy or radiation treatments you – DESPERATELY – need to detox!!!

Consult a functional medicine or naturopathic doctor skilled in detox therapy to help you go through this process.

Purchase a Shower Water Filter

The city water we shower in contains chlorine and fluoride, among other pollutants. Some cities claim their water is "well" water and the best there is – but well water is still required by the FDA to be chlorinated.

Chlorine is a major cancer-causing toxin, especially damaging to women's breasts. Standing in hot, chlorinated water pulsing against the breasts and breathing in the chemical steam – even for ten minutes – is damaging to your body.

People think they will bypass the dangers of contaminated water by putting a filter on the kitchen sink, which is a good idea, but the shower needs a filter too.

Read through this material – and plan your detox.

The best way to successfully traverse a detox protocol is to be *intentional* and *plan ahead*.

1. Choose which detox route you want to take.
2. Schedule when is best to do the detox.
3. Purchase food items ahead of time so day one you are ready to go and know what you are doing.
4. It is highly suggested to make a FOOD & EMOTION JOURNAL. Detoxing brings up emotions because the GI tract is connected via millions of neurotransmitters to the brain. Stored memories and unresolved trauma tend to surface when metabolic fat cells are released during detox and weight loss. Again, be prepared.

Below are the "Do's & Don'ts" of detox; be sure to check out this list and follow these suggestions for the best detox experience. I have listed ways to detox from the simplest daily routine to the more strenuous choices so you can plan ahead and make the best decision for you.

DETOX DO's & DO NOT's

✓ **DO Stay HYDRATED** – drink plenty of clean filtered water and caffeine-free herbal teas throughout the day. Some naturopathic doctors recommend distilled water. You can add fresh squeezed lemon and herbs and/or organic, unfiltered apple cider vinegar for additional cleansing and hydrating affects. The vinegar need only be added 1 or 2 times a day.

A great way to start each day is by drinking warm water with ½ lemon and 1 tablespoon of organic unfiltered apple cider vinegar. You can do this each morning even when you are not actively detoxing. It is a good way to boost the body's natural detoxing mechanisms.

✓ **DO get plenty of NUTRITION** – eat plenty of fresh organic fruits and vegetables, make fresh juice drinks and eat fermented foods like sauerkraut, kimchi and kombucha.

✓ **DO get plenty of REST** – Your body cannot detoxify adequately if you are exhausted. Schedule a good time to detox when you can intentionally calm your life down a bit in order to heal and cleanse.

✓ **DO EXERCISE** – in moderation – no stress, take it easy. Light exercise such as rebounding, walking, deep breathing and stretching to stimulate the lymphatic system.

✓ **DO SWEAT** – the skin is your largest organ, it's vital to sweat out toxins several times each week. A sauna is a great way to do this. Or taking hot steam baths and drinking hot caffeine-free herbal teas. Dry skin brushing before showering is a great way to loosen dead skin cells and stimulate the lymphatic system to eliminate toxins.

- **DO NOT eat BREAD or DAIRY or ANIMAL FOODS**. Meat is acidic and requires a lot of energy to digest. Omit the meat for this detox period and you will achieve greater results. If you tend to be hypoglycemic, you can add an organic vegan protein shake a couple times a day during your detox routine to help with blood sugar spikes. It is helpful for some people to drink this protein shake just before bed to help them sleep more soundly.

- **DO NOT eat SUGAR, SWEETS, or PROCESSED FOODS** – These foods contain chemicals, preservatives, and additives. Stay away from candy and chips, especially. Eat all natural, whole foods, mostly raw if you can.

- **DO NOT STRESS** – Besides making you feel spacy, disconnected and worn down, stress can interfere with proper nutrient absorption. Without certain nutrients, your body will not detox properly.

- **DO NOT** cave into cravings – Make sure to have plenty of fruits and veggies with you at all times so there aren't any temptations to give in to fatty, salty, sugary foods.

- **DO NOT** drink alcohol – Alcohol burdens the liver, and it's counter-productive to burden a body part that you will be detoxing.

- **DO NOT DETOX** if you are pregnant.

- **DO NOT USE SYNTHETIC COSMETICS** – use only pure organic skin care products. Good idea always, but especially during detox.

DETOXING BODY SYSTEMS

The Skin

The skin is the largest eliminating organ of the body, so it's important to take care of your skin on a regular basis, not only during detox. The skin, called the third kidney, eliminates as much waste (by-products and toxins) as your lungs, kidney and bowels.

When you put anything on your skin, on your hair, or on your nails, it seeps into the body because the skin is porous. The cosmetics we women slather on our bodies – everything from conditioners to lipstick – are loaded with toxic chemicals. The Environmental Working Group (EWG), a subsidiary of the Environmental Defense Network puts together a cosmetic database which lists hundreds of thousands of ingredients found in over-the-counter cosmetics. Avoid synthetic products on your skin if at all possible. All of these products contain high levels of cancer and disease causing agents.

Moist, young looking vibrant skin can be achieved with dry skin brushing, Epsom salt rubs and healthy essential oils.

Saunas & Sweating

Sweating is a major way the body eliminates toxins. Hot saunas are an excellent way to sweat and detox. When thyroid function is low, or when one leads a sedentary life, the body does not sweat well. The subcutaneous layers of the skin become clogged or stagnant with toxicity. This causes dry skin, rashes, pimples, dermatitis and dandruff. Sweating is an essential mechanism for getting healthy.

Saunas and steam baths are extremely beneficial. Of course exercise and manual labor are great ways to work up a nice sweat. Got any gardening to do? Great! Feel like a nice early morning run? Hot yoga anyone? Fantastic! Get sweating!

Exercising for Detox

Rebounder:

One of the ways to easily get your lymph system moving is to use a Rebounder. This is a small, individual trampoline. Just hop up and down on the Rebounder for 15 – 20 minutes daily.

Strengthening Core Muscles through Pilates:

A great way to get things moving – and strengthening your body is to do Pilates. Even if you have arthritis or body aches and pains from age or previous injuries, Pilates is a superb way to get your body back into shape. Under the care of a seasoned instructor you can make tremendous headway toward health.

Pilates strengthens the core muscles of your abdomen and torso which also strengthens your immune system. When the immune system is strong the body naturally detoxes with ease.

Yoga:

More people are discovering the health benefits of Yoga. There are beginning classes all the way to expert. Yoga is a great way to stretch and breathe and get all that oxygen into the brain and body. Hot Yoga is a great way to stretch and sweat.

Massage:

Getting a massage is an effective way to help you relax, remove toxins from tissues and helps to get oxygen into every cell of the body.

Acupuncture:

A skilled acupuncturist knows how to help your body heal. When you go in for an examination and health history they understand which body systems are congested and will help you increase the benefits of a detox routine. Also, acupuncture is a great way to enhance the body's natural detox system and help get your body into balance.

A dear friend of mine was suffering from constipation and went to her acupuncturist for help. He put the necessary needles into her hands, and told her to get home fast. She did – and low & behold, her body eliminated beautifully.

Chiropractic Health:

When the spinal cord is out of alignment, the body is out of balance. Blood is restricted from flowing adequately through the nervous system, joints and tissues. If you are suffering from back pain, or elevated hip or knee pain, finding a good chiropractor is 'gold' for helping your body recover health and balance.

Dry Skin Brushing

Dry skin brushing before showering is an excellent way to activate the lymph system and remove dead skin. The skin has many layers, so brushing off the top layer while dry helps the skin breathe, renew itself and release toxins.

Purchase a long-handled vegetable-fiber dry body brush; do not use nylon-bristle on your skin. You can find one at an organic boutique catering to health products or online.

Use the brush daily before showering. Start with your hands and brush vigorously, then up your arms in long strokes toward your heart. The lymph system is the sewer drainage system of the body. Brushing your skin toward your heart helps move stagnant lymphatic fluids out through your liver and kidneys. Brush your feet and legs upward toward your heart. Use the brush to massage your belly and love handles using circular motions. Brush circularly around the knee and elbow joints for some extra stimulation around those joints and ligaments.

Give your body a good upward scrub of love and get those dead skin cells loosened and that lymph system pumping!

Shower Skin-Lymph Massage

One of the ways to continually keep the lymph system moving stagnant fluid out of the body is to use a wash cloth and hold each arm straight over your head one at a time and massage downward with the wash cloth. Do the same with each foot and leg, moving upward toward the heart. A vigorous wash cloth body rub is an excellent way to help with the body's natural detoxification process.

No need for soap *during* the shower massage. Too much soap scrubbed into the body removes the skin's protective microbiome layer. Do not use anti-bacterial soap for the same reason. Your skin's natural microbiome exists as a major part of the immune system. The more natural we keep things, the better the results.

I'm not saying do not use soap to cleanse your body in the shower, what I am saying is while you are vigorously massaging with the wash cloth, just stick with warm water.

Skin Detox Epsom Salt Recipe

This Epsom Salt Massage detox therapy treatment can be done 1 – 3 times a week on a continual basis, not just during detox.

Epsom Salt & Oil Rub Scrub

To really get that dead skin off and get the circulation going, use an Epsom salts – essential oil rub.

Recipe: Use a 1 to 10 ratio – Epson Salt to pure oils of your choice discussed below.

Lemon and citrus essential oils are excellent for detox, but expensive. They can be combined with certified organic oil such as pure fractionated coconut oil, sesame oil, or a certified mineral oil blend from a trusted source such as Dr. John Douillard's *Lymphatic Massage Oil*; http://store.lifespa.com/lymphatic_massage_oil_small.html

1 Small Batch:

- 1 pound Epson Salt
- 1.6 ounces oil

I Large Batch:

- 10 pounds Epson Salt
- 1 pound essential oil mixture

Directions:

1. Wet Epsom salt with clean filtered, structured, or distilled water a little bit at a time until it is the consistency of sand.

2. Add the oil of choice and continue mixing.

3. Put a seat in the shower and without the water running, rub this mixture vigorously and thoroughly over your feet, legs, torso, arms, and even your face. More gently on the face and neck. Rub over every part of your body.

Spend extra time rubbing in circular motions over your joints – and wrists, really rub it in.

4.   Wash it off in your normal shower routine.

This salt – oil scrub has been found to increase the body's circulation by about 10 – 20 times! It helps with arthritis, kidney and liver problems because the skin is the largest cleansing organ in the body. It has even been known to dissolve wrinkles! So get scrubbing and enjoy the benefits.

Drink Lemon Water

Routine for Daily Natural Detox Benefits

Drinking lemon water is perfectly safe to do every morning upon rising, not only during a period of detox. You can mix it up a bit here between these suggestions. The vinegar and baking soda are not pleasant flavors; however they add great healing benefits for the GI tract. Lemon juice also acts to stimulate the liver and get it ready for the day.

1) Drink juice of ½ fresh lemon in 8 oz. clean filtered water at room temperature – or slightly warm water, not hot.

2) For additional health benefits add 1 Tbsp. organic Apple Cider Vinegar to the lemon water.

3) To go to the next step, you can add 1 tsp non-aluminum baking soda to the above mixture. This is especially healing for people suffering from acid indigestion. It will foam a bit and carbonate the mixture.

4) ALSO – for an additional kick start to your liver – you can add a pinch of cayenne pepper.

DAILY JUICING – Natural & Gentle

The next step to kicking up your body's daily detox efforts is to make juicing a regular part of your daily routine. Juice recipes are found in the EDD recipes.

The more raw fruits and vegetables you add to your daily diet, the more alkalizing and detoxing affects your body will enjoy.

Eating a fresh bowl of fruit, or drinking a freshly made fruit smoothie every morning, is a wonderful way to optimize the body's natural cleansing and detoxing efforts.

DETOXING THE COLON

Raw Fruit & Vegetable Juices

The highest nutritional foods on the planet are fresh raw fruits, vegetables, herbs, seaweeds, nuts and seeds. These foods carry the power of life in them. They are full of enzymes, vitamins, minerals, amino acids, antioxidants, simple sugars, water and much more. A diet loaded with fresh, ripe, raw, fruits and vegetables is naturally alkalizing and detoxifying. The more you eat these foods on a regular basis the cleaner your body will be and the more health you will enjoy.

Clean the Colon

Cleaning the colon and *keeping* it clean and operating at optimum condition is vital to preventing cancer and chronic illness. In order to keep the colon clean and functioning properly it is important to eat lots of fiber.

Fiber is a plant-derived carbohydrate that cannot be digested by humans, so it passes through your system relatively intact and it has little or no caloric value. Fiber acts as a natural laxative by increasing stool bulk, which allows stool to pass more readily through the colon.

Fiber in Cruciferous Vegetables: You want to focus on the cruciferous vegetables:

- Arugula
- Bok choy
- Broccoli
- Brussels sprouts
- Cabbage
- Cauliflower
- Collard greens

- Horseradish
- Kale
- Radishes
- Rutabaga
- Turnips
- Watercress
- Wasabi

Organic Psyllium Husk Fiber:

Do not use Metamucil as it is impure and contains additives such as wheat, soy lecithin, sugar, food coloring and more. Use 100% organic psyllium husks.

How to Use Psyllium Husk Fiber:

Psyllium fiber takes some getting used to. It becomes gelatinous immediately upon adding it to liquid. It may trigger the gag reflex, so you want to add it, stir it, and drink it down quickly.

For Daily Use – drink this at night one hour before going to bed.

For Detox – drink this twice a day, morning and evening.

Colon Health Psyllium Husk Recipe

> ➢ 1 heaping tablespoon organic psyllium husk

> ➢ 8 oz. clean, filtered water

> ➢ Option: Add a little bit of pure, fresh squeezed organic grape juice, lemon juice, lime juice, or pineapple juice to the water. Do not use bottled or canned juice.

> ➢ **VERY IMPORTANT – Drink a FULL second 8 ounce glass of water.**

You MUST follow up this mixture with a second glass of water. If you fail to drink this additional glass of water, you are in danger of becoming impacted and causing yourself great abdominal distress.

Vegetable Juice Combinations

Heavy-Metal Detox Combinations

In today's world of heavy toxin load it is important to detox the body from heavy metal build-up using the vegetable combinations found on page 134. These juices can be added to your daily routine and are okay to drink during the EDD.

The following vegetable juice combinations are power packed for the liver, kidneys and adrenals. They are also high in electrolytes, including calcium, magnesium, potassium and sodium. These drinks are rich in chlorophyll for purifying the blood and lymphatic system. Chlorophyll is one of nature's best heavy-metal and chemical detoxifiers.

Add a dash of cayenne pepper to any one of these combinations if desired.

- Carrot + Lemon + Beet + Parsley + Cilantro
- Carrot + Lemon + Beet + Spinach + Cilantro
- Carrot + Lemon + Alfalfa Sprouts + Parsley + Cilantro
- Carrot + Lemon + Spinach + Celery + Parsley + Cilantro
- Wheat grass + Alfalfa sprouts + Cilantro

➤ Adding cabbage and cruciferous vegetables to these combinations is very beneficial for cancer cases. However, this can be bitter and difficult to drink.

Carrots, lemons, cilantro and cayenne pepper bind to heavy metals and help remove them from the body. Cilantro is a critical element to help remove toxins. Some people do not like the taste of cilantro, or say they are allergic to it. So if this is you... maybe using a small amount and working up to a larger amount will help.

Detox Recipe Combinations

This small collection of raw-food recipes will give you some idea of the many simple dishes you can prepare for yourself during detox.

The Master Salad:

Combine any or all of the following:

- Romaine lettuce
- Peas
- Spinach
- Cucumbers
- Olives
- Bell peppers (all colors)
- Onions
- Avocado
- Cabbage (red or white)
- Green beans
- Carrots
- Sweet corn (organic)
- Any dark green leafy vegetable

Make your salad fun and filled with a rainbow of colored vegetables. Use only small amounts of oil-free dressing (more recipes in EDD).

Raw Dressing

- ½ - 1 Avocado
- 2 tsp minced garlic
- ½ cucumber
- ½ cup bell peppers (all colors)
- ¼ small sweet onion
- 1 Tbsp. organic apple cider vinegar; or vinegar of choice

Place ingredients in a blender and blend until a semi-liquid is formed. Pour over your salad as desired.

Guacamole

- 2 cups of diced avocados – skin removed
- 2-3 diced green onions
- Freshly squeezed lemon or lime juice to taste
- ¼ cup chopped bell peppers (optional)
- ½ tsp pink salt (optional)

- 1 tsp cumin
- 1 – 2 Tbsp. chopped parsley & cilantro
- Dash cayenne pepper (optional)

Scoop onto your salad – or use as a dip with an array of fresh vegetables.

Fruit & Melons

Fruit bowls are lovely and delicious – eat whatever organic fruit is in season. Do not eat fruit and melons at the same time. Choose one or the other.

Melons:

Eat melons alone. All varieties are acceptable.

- Watermelon
- Cantaloupe
- Honeydew
- Papaya

> **If you are just leaving the SAD lifestyle behind, it is highly recommended you move on to Chapter 15 and go on the ELIMINATION DETOX DIET before considering a juice or water-only fast.**

Intermittent fasting is a great way to give your body a rest and get rid of toxins.

CHOOSING A "JUICE ONLY" FAST

Going on a juice fast will be invigorating for you if you are already accustomed to periodic fasting routines and want to do a full-body detox to keep things up and running with upgraded health. You can choose to do a juice only fast, or you can do the "combo" juice and vegetable fast described below.

IF you are just coming off the SAD diet, or desire to lose a fair amount of weight, then I do not recommend a juice only fast for you. Your body may trigger the "fight or flight" response, thinking you are heading into a famine, locking down those pounds you want to release. Plus you may be miserable and unable to sustain the decision and end up feeling like a failure.

As Joshua Rosenthal, founder of the Institute of Integrative Nutrition (IIN) says, *"Your body doesn't know when your head makes the decision to go on a diet."*

– JUICE FASTING –

If you are in good health, you can choose to go on a juice only fast for 3 – 14 days. Break the fast (*see directions below*) if it becomes too difficult. Listen to your body and don't push it.

Doing an all fresh fruit and vegetable juice fast is a fantastic way to achieve high levels of anti-oxidants and Alkalizing benefits.

You can also choose to do an all juice fast for three days, and then move into the juice plus raw steamed vegetable fast to elongate the detox benefits without going nuts from hunger. See below for details.

PREPARING FOR AN ALL JUICE FAST

It is best to begin a juice fast gradually.

1. Eliminate all processed, junk & animal food from your diet for at least seven days (or more) before the juice fast.
2. Eat an all raw diet for 2 – 3 days to ease into the total juice fast.
3. Drink lots of clean filtered water. You can add slices of cucumbers, lemons, limes, parsley & cilantro to drinking water for additional cleansing and hydrating benefits.

High Fiber Juicing Method

Using a juicer removes the fiber from fruits and vegetables. One of the ways to increase the fiber in a smoothie and increase the colon cleansing benefits is to prepare your juice using the combination method:

- Juice vegetables; carrots, spinach, kale, celery, parsley etc. in a regular juicer to remove all pulp.
- Then, use high power blender to juice the fruit; apples, peeled oranges, peeled lemons, strawberries, blue berries, bananas, watermelon, etc.
- Add the blended fruit to the juiced vegetables for a delicious potent detox elixir.

TWO POWERHOUSE JUICES

Two of the best single-fruit juices are grape juice and apple juice. These will supply loads of calcium while they clean the liver and kidneys and feed the nerve and glandular system.

GRAPE JUICE RECIPE:

Use ONLY *organic* grapes as grapes are one of the "dirty dozen" pesticide filled foods.

- Juice the grapes, seeds and stems in a high-power blender until thoroughly liquefied and strain.

Effects: Tumor buster, lymph stimulation, free-radical eliminator, toxicity removal (including heavy metals and minerals), strengthens the heart and vascular system.

APPLE JUICE RECIPE:

Use ONLY *organic* apples as apples are one of the "dirty dozen" pesticide filled foods.

- Juice the apples with skin, seeds and stems in a high-power blender until thoroughly liquefied and strain.

Effects: Enzyme-rich juice aids digestion, supplies amino acids, eliminates free-radicals and strengthens the body.

These juices can be used on a juice fast alone – using only this juice if you desire. Or, intersperse these juices with other fruit juices if desired.

– INSTRUCTIONS FOR BREAKING A JUICE FAST –

!!! IMPORTANT !!!!!

If you decide to go on a total juice fast even for a short period of time – it is VITAL to add solid foods *slowly* back into your diet to prevent your body from triggering the 'fight or flight' response. If you adhere to the following food re-introduction instructions, your body will benefit from your fasting efforts and continue to heal.

1. After a liquid juice fast, begin by adding fresh fruit. Eat melons alone; and only 1 – 3 types of raw fresh fruit at a time. Don't over load yourself, take it easy. Add fresh fruit several times during the day on day 1 and day 2 when breaking the fast.

1. On days 3 and 4 after breaking the fast; add raw or steamed vegetables. Again, be careful not to overload your digestive tract. Boiling vegetables into a nice soup is soothing and satisfying. It's okay to season the soup with herbs of your choice including garlic, oregano, rosemary, thyme, turmeric, onion, parsley and cilantro.

2. On day five introduce small meals of fresh organic ingredients back into your diet and see how you feel.

JUICE & VEGETABLE COMBINATION FAST

Breakfast - *Choose one*

1. Fruit
2. Melon

Pick any single or combination of fruits or melons that you like.

Between Meal Juice

Drink an 8 oz. to 10 oz. glass of freshly juiced vegetable or fruit juice.

Lunch and Dinner - *Choose one*

1. Large salad, with a side of vegetables: Steamed or raw vegetable soup, water or vegetable broth sautéed stir fry medley; no tomato. Use the list of cruciferous vegetables found earlier in this chapter.

2. Fruit

3. Melon

Chapter 15
The Elimination Detox Diet
Let's Get Started on Our New Road to Health!

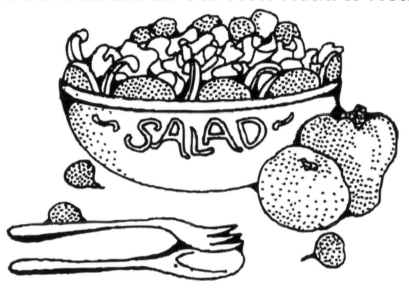

Your new healthy upgraded lifestyle begins here with the Elimination Detox Diet (EDD). The EDD is the gentlest, most effective way to get started on sustainable healthy lifestyle changes. The key is to commit and stick with it. YOU CAN DO IT!

THE ELIMINATION DETOX DIET (EDD)

As we have learned, GMO's, pesticides, food additives and chemicals are wreaking havoc in people's digestive tract and causing allergic reactions from eating certain difficult to digest foods.

We will determine which food or foods may be causing the most damage by going on the EDD.

The EDD removes specific foods that may be causing your Body Speak Symptoms. These acidic and difficult to digest foods include alcohol, animal foods, caffeine, corn, dairy, eggs, fish, gluten, shellfish, soy and nuts. This list may seem daunting – but I have included a step by step meal guide and delicious recipes that will leave you satisfied and never hungry. Your body will LOVE you for it – and reward you with detoxing, releasing unwanted weight and renewed energy.

> **Following this EDD protocol will empower you to regain control of your appetite and strengthen you to leave unhealthy habits behind.**

The EDD removes specific foods *for a period of time* – minimum of 21 days – and observes how the body reacts. After the elimination phase, foods are reintroduced one at a time to see whether the symptoms resurface, signaling which specific foods are the issue. ***Keeping a food diary is suggested to record any adverse physical or emotional reactions.***

An elimination diet is not a "cure" but rather an odyssey of discovery. By eliminating the foods that most commonly cause digestion issues, we are able to locate the specific foods that are causing discomfort and damaging the body.

Elimination Diet – is Naturally Detoxifying

The EDD is naturally detoxing because removing foods that are particularly difficult to digest and eating clean whole foods frees up energy the body needs to get rid of toxins stored in fat cells.

Gentle Detox – What to Expect

If you are a heavy caffeine user removing caffeine may cause headaches and the shakes. Try cutting back gradually the week or two heading into this diet. Prepare ahead and think about it. Green tea has a small amount of caffeine, but it is permissible during the EDD. Drinking green tea may be a way of helping to break the caffeine habit and it is detoxing and healthy.

Also, for heavy sugar users, cravings will surface for the first few days, but after that you should level out and enjoy the program successfully.

Some people suffer no side effects from this gentle detox, but it is good to prepare for some discomfort at the beginning.

Here are some of the symptoms you may experience for a short period of time.

Detox Symptoms:

- Cravings
- Dizziness
- Digestive upset
- Exhaustion
- Fluid retention
- Getting sick – or flu like symptoms
- Headaches
- Irritability
- Irritable bowel from runny to constipated
- Lethargy
- Mood swings
- PMS
- Skin breakouts; acne
- Sore red or stinging eyes
- Sleep disturbance; waking between 2-4 am – especially waking hot
- Sinus congestion, sneezing, allergy type symptoms

Here's the GOOD NEWS – EXPECT AWESOME RESULTS!!!

- ✓ Clear skin
- ✓ No headaches
- ✓ Lose 10 lbs. *(or more)*
- ✓ Sugar cravings gone
- ✓ Reduce severe allergies
- ✓ Cooking more – fun!
- ✓ More energy

3 Meals a Day – No Snacks

Eat three meals per day – and eat to satisfaction, do not worry about calories. While eating the foods acceptable on this diet protocol, you will lose weight naturally and detox gently. This is not a depravation diet, but rather a food sensitivity elimination diet.

Cutting out snacks and aiming for three meals a day may sound hard to do, but it is worth trying and here's why.

Many of us have trained our bodies to rely on snacks or small meals every few hours or less. This tells the body there is a constant supply of energy coming in, so there is no reason to burn stored fat.

Burning stored fat is important even if you aren't trying to lose weight. Our fat cells store toxins, so when the body utilizes stored fat it gently removes toxins and helps the body maintain a healthy, balanced weight.

How to Transition to 3 Meals a Day

If you are used to snacking or have adopted a diet of frequent small meals, eating three meals a day will require transition. Here are some tips to ease in:

- Start with four meals a day with no snacks in between and gradually work towards three meals a day.
- Make each meal psychologically satisfying by stopping, sitting down, and enjoying each bite.
- Eat enough food at breakfast to carry you through to lunch.
- Eat a big, warm, satisfying lunch between the hours of 10am and 2pm. It is believed that lunch should be the biggest meal of the day. Eat enough to carry you through to supper.
- Eat a light, early supper – think of supper as 'supplemental' to your midday meal, rather than a big stand-alone meal. That said; eat enough supper to carry you through the night until breakfast without hunger. If you are not sleeping well, it may mean you need to eat more at supper.

BLOOD SUGAR BALANCING

Blood sugar crashes are not uncommon in the first days of the EDD, especially if you are shooting for three meals a day with no snacks. After living a lifestyle that relies heavily on snacks and/or small, frequent meals, three meals a day can be a bit of a shock.

You may experience a crash quite suddenly, even after having done well for a few days. Stress, not-quite-right timing of meals, or not eating enough at your previous meal can all be insidious reasons for a blood sugar crash.

Keeping your blood sugar balance is vital. The important thing is to know what to do when a blood sugar crash happens – and not to panic. This does not mean you failed at the diet, or that the diet should be over.

What to Do If You Experience a Blood-Sugar Crash:

The first thing to do is have a snack. I know I just said no snacks, but blood sugar dips are scary and unpleasant.

Have a nonfat healthy snack, like fruit or carrots, or eat an orange. Green apples are a great way to keep detoxing and boost blood sugar. When you are out and about, take green apples with you.

The Second Thing to Do is to Add Protein to Your Future Meals

Quinoa is an excellent protein source and has more protein than rice. Try building your next meal around quinoa. If you hate quinoa, beans and broccoli which are high in vegetable protein can be substituted.

You can add a small (8 ounce) organic non-soy, non-dairy based protein shake to your next meal and with each midday meal thereafter (or each meal, if you need) until you feel your blood sugar stabilize. It can be whey, pea, hemp, or rice protein, but try for a concentrate rather than an isolate (look for this in the Nutrition Facts on the label.)

If you are Hypoglycemic, Diabetic and / or Low Thyroid:

Adding grains to your diet may cause low energy, and blood sugar spikes and crashes. If this is the case, then add a palm sized serving of *organic* white chicken or *organic* white turkey meat to your next meal and each midday meal thereafter.

Preparing for the EDD

It will be easier for you if you head into the EDD prepared. The best way to do this is to remove the following foods and begin eating organic home-cooked meals and salads for 1 – 2 weeks before starting the diet.

- Alcohol - *if you are used to drinking wine with dinner or daily, try to ween off with organic red wine then taper off to be alcohol free during the EDD*
- Caffeine - *if you are a heavy caffeine consumer begin to cut back gradually*
- Fast Food
- Junk Food
- Restaurant Food
- Sugar
- In-between meals snacks

Take a Food Inventory

Now is the time to go through your refrigerator, freezer and pantry and get rid of everything that is not going to help you make a clean start in living a healthy lifestyle.

Read the labels of every bottle of BBQ sauce, condiments, etc. Look for sugar content, if sugar is listed in the first three ingredients, throw it out. And, if there are any ingredients you do not recognize as human food, like ingredients that you can't even pronounce, throw it out.

Begin to think 'clean' and 'healthy.' What does this mean to you? What changes are you willing to make for you? Be honest, now is the time to evaluate what food means to you and how much it may be controlling you.

Ponder your relationship to food. What is food to you? Comfort? Entertainment? Obsession? It is important to understand what is the driving force behind the food choices we make each day.

Check Out the Food List, Recipes & Prepare for Elimination Diet

Take a look at the **Shopping List** in the next chapter and browse through the recipes. Begin to plan your grocery shopping to officially begin the EDD on the date you've selected.

The Crowding Out Method

Be creative and try foods you have never cooked before. The new foods you love, add to your regular food rotation – and the foods you do not care for, well now you know!

The key to crowding out – is to replace the old with the new. Eat until you are satisfied at each meal. There is no need to feel hungry or deprived. Deprivation will lead to binge eating, giving in to bad habits, discouragement and giving up.

The recipes in this book are designed to be your launching pad in the kitchen. You can easily enjoy nourishing and delicious meals that meet the healing and detox guidelines for the EDD. Hopefully, you will enjoy these recipes so much you will add them into your weekly meal rotation after this program.

A healthy diet means most meals are home-cooked. This may be something of a challenge for you at the beginning, but do the best you can – and don't stress! Make it simple, easy and enjoyable. Choose the recipes that appeal to you and add your own personal chef flair!

Feel free to mix and match all the acceptable foods listed here. The best rule of thumb is to eat what is fresh, in season and organic.

EMOTIONAL CHECK- IN & SELF- INQUIRY

On this journey, when your body releases fat cells, there is an emotional and psychological component. Metabolizing fat provides a great opportunity to face and move through emotional patterns that may have a history of holding you back from greater joy or from realizing your full potential. Like some toxins, molecules of emotion have also been found to be stored in our fat cells. This includes fat cells in the brain and in other tissues of the body *(Pert, C. Molecules of Emotion, 1997. Simon and Schuster. New York).*

Detoxing Emotions

When fat metabolism really kicks in, use a journal to document how you feel and what emotional issues and opportunities are arising for you during the detox. As you begin to de-stress and these emotions begin to surface, you will likely feel more sensitive and maybe a touch more irritable. If we can recognize them as such, these emotional moments are opportunities to change our emotional patterns by responding differently.

When emotions arise, choose awareness and acceptance, and look to see what these emotions are connected to. Why did they arise? Journal through these emotions and learn how to respond, not react, and you will be able to experience a different outcome that will empower you and your healing journey.

INTENTION AND AWARENESS

Primary Food & Secondary Food

There is more to life than the food on your plate! Food is actually secondary and all the rest of life is primary.

The danger with food is – it is *entertaining*, distracting, fun and social. Food changes the mood pretty quickly so it can easily become a 'comfort' coping mechanism. The goal is to remove our emotional attachment to food and realize food is nothing more than a way to provide nutrition to our body. Just like putting gasoline in a car. Remember – eat to live, don't live to eat.

There is a reason behind every choice you make, and when you become aware of those reasons, you will have the power to change your choices. When you choose to nurture yourself, your life and your body, your life will take a major turn toward joy, health, balance and fulfillment.

When you grow in awareness of your daily choices, you gain power in your life. When you allow something – or someone – outside of yourself to control you, like toxic relationships, or the food you crave and give into – then you begin to feel powerless and out of control; which leads to a downward spiral of victim thinking and accepting helplessness.

Feeling helpless is dangerous because it leads to out-of-control – act out – behavior. Which in turn, leads to the inevitable conclusion; *"Oh what's the use, nothing ever changes. I might as well go out and ..."* fill in the blank.

Giving in to binges and the negative behaviors you hate will never make you happy. Let alone empower you to unlock the amazing, powerful person you are! There is only one you. You were sent to this earth with a purpose that only you can fulfill.

Using Sweeteners

We all have a tendency toward having a "sweet tooth" which causes cravings, and giving in to sugar cravings can trigger eating binges.

It is advised to stay away from all sweeteners during the EDD; even natural sweeteners like stevia. This gives your body a chance to detox from the sweet taste. Even if you work hard to balance the blood sugar during the diet, a lingering addiction to the sweet taste can undermine lasting results.

Take this time to ween yourself off the need for sweet. It is possible to slay your sweet tooth and be free of sugar cravings once and for all. I have done this – and let me tell you – I LOVE not having sugar cravings!

FOOD RE-INTRODUCTION – *Very Important!*

If you enjoy the results of eating soy-free, gluten-free and plant-based – feel free to do so for as long as you are thriving. You can find lots of fun and delicious recipes by searching "Gluten-free Vegan." Also, searching "Raw" will serve up some incredibly creative and delicious fare.

AFTER 21- DAY EDD

Once the 21-days are complete, foods are reintroduced, *one at a time*. Choose only one food from the eliminated food list and try it for 3 – 4 days. It may take that long for food sensitivity symptoms to return which is why it is important to wait before re-introducing a second food. Food intolerance symptoms include sinus/mucous buildup, sneezing/allergy type symptoms, indigestion, heartburn, nausea, cramps, headaches, fatigue, constipation or diarrhea, among others.

Keep track of how you feel, if symptoms flare up, remove this food from your diet. If symptoms do not return in 3 – 4 days after reintroduction, this food is safe to add back into your diet. Now it is time to reintroduce the next eliminated food item and continue the process.

Food sensitivities are a result of having an "immune response." Remember when we talked about inflammation and the 'adaptive' immune system? Immune cells have memory that lasts for months and even years. Twenty-one days is not long enough to fully recover gut health – however – 21 days is long enough to get a reaction when you reintroduce a food your body isn't prepared to handle yet.

Food Allergies vs Food Sensitivities

When we are allergic to a food the body has a permanent adverse reaction. This food cannot be eaten again.

Food sensitivity may simply be a digestive issue for now, but once the gut is healed these foods will no longer create adverse reactions in the body. This could take months to even years depending on the severity of gut damage.

The good news is, we can heal our digestion through eating clean, whole foods, fruits and vegetables, probiotics and fermented foods. When we give our bodies the nutrients it needs, it can heal and recover from food sensitivities.

Chapter 16
EDD Acceptable Foods
Shopping & Cooking Guides

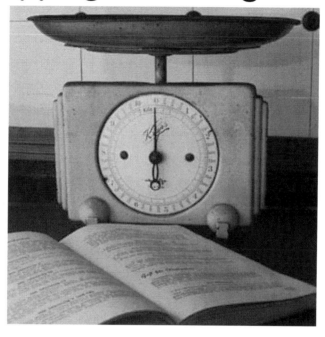

This chapter includes diet guidelines, acceptable food lists and cooking guides to complete the 21-Day Elimination Detox Diet. Pre-planning is vital for success – have everything ready to go on day one.

> **The best way to change your diet and lifestyle is to focus on all the wonderful food choices you *do* have – rather than on the foods you are choosing to eliminate.**

Plant-based Vegan Tastes vs. SAD Animal Food Tastes

Let's face it, eating chemically enhanced, high salt, fat and sugary meals has set our taste buds up for certain expectations. We want that 'bam' of sweet, or that 'jolt' of salty seasoned chips, or the satisfaction of biting into a fat, juicy cheeseburger. The EDD tastes and textures are NOT the same. Taste buds need time to adjust. Choose a health mindset and your body and taste buds will catch up.

Whether you are choosing to add more plant-based meals to your life, or planning to go full steam ahead into the EDD, the transition will take time to adjust. Animal based meals are very different than plant-based meals. It is easy to plan a meal around chicken or a steak, but finding that satisfying 'base' in vegan cooking is the challenge. If you are totally new to considering a plant based diet – as I was in the beginning – it can be overwhelming. I am a skilled home cook and entertainer. I love to wow my family and friends with delectable satisfying foods. When we first started eating like this I used my entertainment filter to judge each meal. Would I serve this to family & friends? Would I order this in a restaurant? If the answer was yes, it was added to our meal rotation.

Go into this positive, thoughtful, and planning ahead. Don't bite off more than you can chew, or you will get discouraged and go get a burger! Be patient with yourself and have a 'marathon' mentality – not a 'sprint' short-term attitude.

Maintain an open mind, experiment and don't give up! You can do this.

> ➢ **Important**: Plant based meals are delicious – *but* – they are not animal based so the textures and tastes are different. A vegan pizza is NOT going to have the same taste and texture as a regular pizza. Broth sautéed vegetables have a different texture than oil sautéed. Your taste buds will adjust. Soon, you will be detecting the taste of oil and other additives in the food you eat out and preferring your own home cooking!

Elimination Detox Diet Food Guide

ALL fruits, vegetables and grains listed here are acceptable.

FRUITS:

Fruits marked with (*) are extra cleansing

As a general rule, eat fruit separately, do not combine with other foods. If you choose to make one of the overnight oatmeal breakfast recipes; a small amount of fruit is permitted in the oatmeal. Otherwise, eat separately.

Eat melons by themselves.

Fruits:	jack fruit	blueberries	plums
apples	kiwi	cherries	strawberries
apricots	*mangos	cranberries	*tangerines
*bananas	nectarines	*grapefruit	
blackberries	papayas	guava	**Melon**
coconuts (ripe)	peaches	*lemons	cantaloupe
dragon fruit	pears (*ripe*)	*limes	honey dew
*figs	persimmons	*oranges	watermelon
*grapes	raspberries	pineapples	papaya

VEGETABLES:

Vegetables marked with (*) are extra cleansing

artichokes	chives	kohlrabi	rutabaga
*beets	*cilantro	hot peppers	seaweed
broccoli	*chilies	leeks	spinach
baby greens	collard greens	lettuce	sprouts
bamboo shoots	cucumber	mushrooms	squash
beets	dandelion	mustard	*sweet
bell peppers	greens	greens	potatoes
bok choy	endive	okra	Swiss chard
broccoli rabe	escarole	olives	*tomatoes
*Brussel	eggplant	onions	turnips
sprouts	fennel	parsley	watercress
*carrots	ginger	parsnip	yams
cabbage	green beans	potatoes	*winter squash
cauliflower	green peas	*pumpkins	zucchini
celery	jicama	radishes	
chicory	kale	red leaf chicory	

ACCEPTABLE GLUTEN-FREE GRAINS

- Amaranth
- Brown & white rice
- Buckwheat
- Millet

- Oats
- Quinoa
- Sorghum
- Teff

Corn Meal is also gluten-free but for the sake of the EDD, we are eliminating corn. Just know in the future corn does not have gluten. Eat only non-GMO organic corn.

Sweetener:

- Raw unfiltered honey
- Pure maple syrup

Try to avoid sweetener on the EDD. There are a couple recipes included here that use 1 – 2 tsp honey or maple syrup, this scant amount is permissible in these recipes.

Unsweetened Non-Dairy Milk Substitutes:

- Almond milk
- Coconut milk

- Hemp milk
- Rice milk

Read labels; may contain hidden sugar & preservatives.

Beverages:

- Green Tea *(has low level of caffeine but permitted because of anti-cancer health benefits)*
- Distilled or clean, filtered water
- Herbal tea (non-caffeinated)
- Homemade carbonated water; add fresh squeezed lemon & lime, mint, or slices of cucumber if desired.

Oil*: Do not use oil on the EDD. After the EDD use small amounts of coconut oil to sauté vegetables and for baked foods; organic olive oil can be used in small amounts in salad dressings. It is not advisable to cook with olive oil.

> ➤ *There is growing concern in the health community of the damaging effects of oil in the body; even coconut oil. Oil is an isolate, meaning it is stripped of all nutritional value, and coats the inner cells of our body.*

> ➤ ** On the EDD, you can add 1 tsp toasted sesame oil to Asian flavored foods and sauces. The flavor is awesome and this scant amount is not an issue.*

Healthy Fats:

Avocado
Seeds; chia, hemp, pumpkin, sesame, sunflower
Nuts are not permitted on the EDD.

***After* EDD** – Nuts and nut butters such as almond, cashew and organic peanut butter are healthy fats. Nut butters are a great way to add creamy texture to soups and stews.

Vinegars:

- Apple cider vinegar
- Balsamic vinegar
- Red or white wine vinegar
- Rice vinegar
- Raspberry

How Much Salt?

Avoid table salt. It is bleached and contains other chemical additives. Enjoy small amounts of healthier alternatives, such as pink Himalayan, Kosher or sea salt.

INTERNALLY 'COOK' YOUR FOOD WITH WATER

Drink WATER before each meal.

Drink about 8 oz. clean, filtered water about 10-15 minutes before each meal. This helps the stomach prepare to 'cook' the food you eat. It also helps reduce acid indigestion and gives your body a good head-start in preparing to absorb all the nutrients possible from your meal.

We took Prilosec daily for years to combat heartburn. Now that we eat mostly plant-based organic, and drink 8 oz. of water before each meal, we no longer suffer from heartburn and do not take antacids or heartburn medication.

Avoid Processed Foods

Processed foods include not only boxed or ready-made meals found in the center grocery and freezer aisles, but also pastas, breads, gluten-free foods, tortillas, cookies, candies, cold cuts, breakfast cereals, canned fruits and vegetables, potato chips, vegetable oils, soda & energy drinks, even if labeled "organic," "natural," or "whole-grain."

Asian rice noodles and 100% buckwheat soba noodles are acceptable in small amounts while on the EDD when eaten with lots of vegetables. Keep portion size to ½ cup and only once or twice in *a week*, not every day as detox benefits will be impeded.

Organic Brown-Rice Cakes: The only 'processed' foods allowed during the 21-day EDD are – organic brown-rice cakes; slightly salted is okay. Do not eat the 'flavored' rice cakes. Keep it to no more than two a day. Rice cakes crumbled over a salad adds a nice crunch. Rice cakes dipped in salsa & oil-free hummus coupled with a platter of fresh crisp vegetables for dipping makes a refreshing and satisfying light meal.

> ➤ **TIP**: In order to detox – the more fresh, raw fruits and vegetables you eat the better.

Eat in Peace & Enjoy Every Bite!

HEALTHY COOKING GUIDELINES

Here are some simple, healthy cooking instructions and guidelines to follow on the EDD.

- NO MICROWAVE COOKING -

"SADLY," *(pun intended)* microwave energy alters the structural integrity of food removing all nutritional value. Do not use a microwave. Ever.

> **Feel free to be creative with acceptable food choices.**
> **There is a lot to choose from – let your creativity flow.**
> **Have fun and experiment with new foods.**

RAW Soup – Excellent for healing and detoxing.

You can put your favorite vegetables and seasonings into a high-powered blender and blend until the mixture becomes hot - approximately 6 - 10 minutes, depending on the blender. Just lift the lid and see the steam escape, and you'll know it is ready. This is warm and comforting and still considered raw - because the mixture does not reach a cooking temperature. This is a nutritious and detoxing way to make soup.

How to Enjoy Greens

- Many people find greens more palatable when they parboil them for 2-5 minutes in a shallow pan of water, then strain them. This removes the bitter tasting compounds.

- Lemon juice helps greens taste less bitter.

- When you steam greens for 8-10 minutes and blend then into a soup, the micro-nutrients (minerals and vitamins) become more bio-available.

- Collards make a great replacement for tortillas – simply add some rice and beans (or filling of your choice) with sprouts inside a collard leaf and fold like a wrap. You can keep the collard wrap raw or steam it briefly.

- Romaine leaves make a great wrap or "boat" for tasty fillings.

How to Water or Vegetable Broth Sauté

- Instead of sautéing vegetables in oil, use water or low sodium organic vegetable broth. Sauté them by bringing a small amount of water or broth to a fast boil in saucepan, then add your vegetables and sauté them as you would in oil. Add small amounts of water or broth if needed until vegetables reach desired consistency.

- The texture of water sautéed vegetables is 'lighter' than when using oil. This may take a little bit of getting used to, but once you do, you will not miss the oil. In fact, the flavors of the vegetables and grains will be more savory and delicious without oil.

How to Make Vegetable Broth

Commercially processed broths and stocks contain a great deal of processed sodium and other additives we are trying to avoid during the EDD. Please consider making your own vegetable broth as a base for soups, stews, and cooking grains. It's very easy to do and will add more nutrition and flavor.

Homemade Sodium-Free Vegetable Broth

Yields: 4-5 servings

Use this stock any time a recipe calls for water when cooking soups, sauces, or whole grains.

- 3 stalks celery, roughly chopped
- 3 carrots, roughly chopped
- 4 tsp garlic, minced
- 2 onions, roughly chopped (or leeks, shallots, or green onions)

- 2-3 cups water
- 2-3 cups vegetable scraps (optional)
- 2 bay leaves

Stove top method:

1. In a large soup pot, combine all the ingredients
2. Cover. Bring to a boil. Reduce heat to low and simmer for at least 45 minutes (or up to a few hours).
3. Let cool, then strain.

Slow cooker method:

1. Combine all the ingredients in a slow cooker. Cook on low for 8-10 hours or on high for 5-6 hours.
2. Let cool, then strain.

Asian-style broth: Add ginger and/or lemongrass.

Italian-style: Add tomato and sprigs of thyme, rosemary, sage, oregano, and/or basil.

Refrigerate or freeze extra broth. Vegetable broth can keep for 1 week in the fridge or 6 months in the freezer. You can freeze in ice cube trays, plastic freezer bags, or containers such as Tupperware® or Mason jars (leave room for the liquid to expand in the container as it freezes).

> **Tip: A Note about Vegetable Scraps**: You can make stock exclusively from scraps! Collect and freeze scraps to enhance nutrition and flavor of your broth. Save scraps such as mushroom stems, cilantro stems, celery leaves, ribs from leafy green veggies, corn cobs, asparagus ends, and the peels from garlic, onions, beets, carrots, potatoes, etc. Do not save anything old or moldy. Avoid cruciferous vegetables, such as cauliflower, cabbage, broccoli or Brussels sprouts, as they tend to make the broth bitter.

Soaking & Cooking Grains

To improve digestibility, try soaking whole grains. When possible, soak all whole grains for at least an hour, ideally overnight. Drain and rinse before cooking.

This includes *steel-cut oats* for oatmeal. Try to remember to soak them the night before when you are planning on making *steel-cut* oatmeal for breakfast.

Grains Basic Cooking Directions:

Remember: One cup of dry grains yields 2–4 servings.

Gluten-Free Grains Cooking Chart

1 Cup	Water	Cooking Time
Amaranth	3 cups	30 minutes
Brown rice	2 cups	45–60 minutes
Buckwheat (aka kasha)	2 cups	20–30 minutes
Cornmeal (aka polenta)	3 cups	20 minutes
Millet	2 cups	30 minutes
Oats (whole oats)	3 cups	45–60 minutes
Oatmeal (rolled oats)	2 cups	45–60 minutes
Quinoa	2 cups	15–20 minutes
Wild rice	4 cups	60 minutes

1. Measure the grain, check for bugs or unwanted materials, and rinse in cold water using a fine mesh strainer.
2. Soak grains for one to eight hours to soften, increase digestibility, and eliminate phytic acid. Drain grains and discard the soaking water.
3. Add grains to recommended amount of water and bring to a boil.
4. Reduce heat, cover, and simmer for the suggested amount of time without stirring during the cooking process.

Soaking or Sprouting Beans

Always soak beans for at least 8 hours, or overnight. This helps with the digestibility. Soaking beans for 24 – 48 hours will 'sprout' the beans. They do not begin to grow, but this process **renders** them even easier to digest.

ALL BEANS are acceptable on the EDD.

Quick-Soak Dried Bean Method

When time is of the essence – and you want beans for a meal, but did not remember to soak them ahead, use this method.

1. Rinse and drain your choice of dried beans. Place beans in Dutch oven or large soup pot and cover with water to about one inch over beans. Sprinkle with about 1 tsp of pink Himalayan, Kosher or sea salt and bring to a boil.
2. Boil for one full minute. Turn off heat, cover and soak for 60 minutes.
3. Drain water, rinse and proceed with recipe.

Endless Variations: Veggies, Grains, and Beans

Plan meals for a week at a time:

Check out the *Culinary Spices from Around the World* table on the next page, read through the recipes – and understand how to soak and cook grains and beans and plan your menu.

You can create multitudes of satiating meals by combining different variations of your favorite vegetables, grains, beans and spices.

Mix it up with different spices; Italian, Mexican, Indian, and Asian. There is no limit to the creativity you can produce with these ingredients.

> **Choose a non-gluten grain:** Amaranth, buckwheat, millet, quinoa, brown or white long grain rice – or organic gluten-free (GF) grain blend.

> **Choose your legume or beans**: Small beans are easiest to digest, but all beans are permissible; adzuki, lentils, mung, split yellow mung, black, black-eyed peas, cannellini, garbanzo, fava, kidney, lima, navy or pinto.

> **Choose your vegetables**: Enjoy any and all seasonal vegetables steamed, broth sautéed, raw or in a salad.

> **Choose Flavor Profile:** Select what you are in the mood for and design your meal around these flavor profiles.

> Be sure to include plenty of raw salads, fresh vegetables, leafy greens and green apples to your meals every day.

Culinary Spices from Around the World

INDIAN

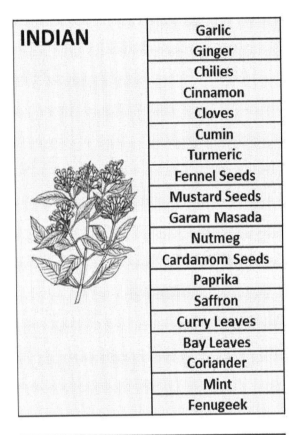

Garlic
Ginger
Chilies
Cinnamon
Cloves
Cumin
Turmeric
Fennel Seeds
Mustard Seeds
Garam Masada
Nutmeg
Cardamom Seeds
Paprika
Saffron
Curry Leaves
Bay Leaves
Coriander
Mint
Fenugeek

MEXICAN

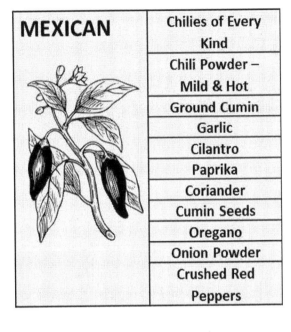

Chilies of Every Kind
Chili Powder – Mild & Hot
Ground Cumin
Garlic
Cilantro
Paprika
Coriander
Cumin Seeds
Oregano
Onion Powder
Crushed Red Peppers

ASIAN

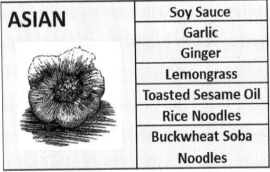

Soy Sauce
Garlic
Ginger
Lemongrass
Toasted Sesame Oil
Rice Noodles
Buckwheat Soba Noodles

ITALIAN

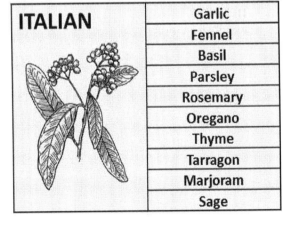

Garlic
Fennel
Basil
Parsley
Rosemary
Oregano
Thyme
Tarragon
Marjoram
Sage

HOMEMADE JAMAICAN JERK SPICE

This is a great spice mix to have on hand when you are making a veggie stir-fry, or looking to kick-up the flavor of soups or stews. Double or quadruple recipe and keep stored in air-tight glass container. Keeps indefinitely.

Yields: Approximately ¼ cup

Ingredients:

- 1 Tbsp. garlic powder
- 2 – 3 tsp cayenne pepper
- 2 tsp onion powder
- 2 tsp dried thyme
- 2 tsp dried parsley
- 2 tsp coconut sugar
- 2 tsp sea salt
- 1 tsp sweet or smoked paprika
- 1 tsp ground allspice
- ½ tsp crushed black pepper
- ½ tsp dried crushed red pepper
- ½ tsp ground nutmeg
- ¼ tsp ground cinnamon

BASIC VEGAN SHOPPING LIST:

Here is a list of the basic items you need in your pantry to embark on this eating plan. Choose organic, certified non-GMO products.

- ✓ Almond milk, unsweetened
- ✓ Almond flour
- ✓ Assortment of organic canned beans
- ✓ Assortment dried beans
- ✓ Better than Bouillon Organic Vegetable Base*
- ✓ Organic Brown & white rice
- ✓ Organic Coconut flour
- ✓ Coconut milk, unsweetened
- ✓ Flax seed
- ✓ Garlic, large jar minced
- ✓ Ginger, jar or tube minced
- ✓ Honey raw, organic
- ✓ Lentils
- ✓ Liquid Aminos *(soy sauce alternative)*

- ✓ Low-sodium organic soy sauce
- ✓ Maple syrup, pure
- ✓ Nutritional Yeast
- ✓ Pink Himalayan salt
- ✓ Organic Apple-cider vinegar
- ✓ Sunflower seeds
- ✓ Tapioca Starch
- ✓ TruRoots** Organic Grain Blend
- ✓ TruRoots** Organic Rice Blend
- ✓ Toasted Sesame Seed oil
- ✓ Vegetable Broth; organic low-sodium
- ✓ Vinegar; balsamic, rice, red & white wine; *all* acceptable

* **Better than Bouillon Organic Vegetable Base** is a delicious – must have – seasoning for vegetarian dishes. It can be found at Sprouts and other health food retailers. Just add 1 tablespoon of this tasty base to any soup, sauce or stew for a rich depth of flavor.

****TruRoots** is a quality company who has developed organic, certified non-GMO sprouted wheat and grain products. Sometimes you can find their products at Costco, Sprouts, or your health food retailers. Or, you can find them online, here is a link to the company, you can check out their products and order some up for your own pantry. http://www.truroots.com/products/truroots-accents.

Spices: Check out the *Culinary Spices From Around the World* for spice suggestions and pick up the ones that look interesting that you do not already have in your spice cupboard. Have fun and be creative with seasoning and spices.

KITCHEN TOOLS

INSTANT- POT – Pressure Cooker & Crockpot

The modern-age miracle – "INSTANT-POT" saves *hours* in the kitchen! This wonder of culinary engineering cooks perfect brown rice in 22 minutes (*normally 45-50)*. It is a rice cooker, a pressure cooker, and a crockpot. It works like a dream to speed up your meals and brings a level of convenience vital for today's busy home cooks.

There are several brands on the market. Check it out and seriously consider picking up one of these – or add it to your Christmas list. It is worth it. With a basic list of ingredients on hand from the above list, and fresh veggies in the fridge, a tasty, wholesome meal can be on the table in about 30 - 45 minutes. Unheard of when cooking beans and lentils from scratch.

Food Processors

> A coffee grinder is helpful to grind grains into powders for baking and making cereals.

> We use a "Ninja" food processor to easily mince onion, herbs, and vegetables for soups. Also useful for grinding nuts and making nut butter after the EDD.

> Heavy duty blender for juices, soups, and smoothies.

Body Speak!

Chapter 17

SAD Recovery Bootcamp

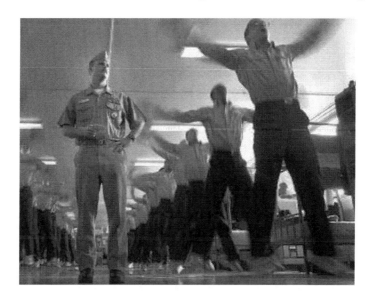

Successfully Navigating the Busy Work Week

Fast-food lunches? *Strike you're out!*

Drive-thru on the way home from work? *No more!*

Transitioning from SAD to a healthy lifestyle means that fast food, drive-through's and junk food are no longer part of your life.

I call this boot camp because you are learning how to make significant and sustainable changes that will revolutionize your health. This is accomplished as painlessly as possible by arming you with delicious and satisfying recipes and a meal plan that can be modified to fit into any busy schedule. As you plan ahead and make these changes you are well on your way to your new healthy lifestyle!

Culinary tools necessary to achieve optimal success:

1) Heavy-Duty Blender
2) Juicer
3) Instant-Pot Pressure Cooker, Crockpot or, regular Crockpot – a must!
4) Large BPA-free plastic travel container for smoothies
5) Glass air tight containers for meals on the go
6) Thermos for hot & cold meals
7) Insulated lunch box travel container

Basic Plan of Execution:

1. Plan meals for the week.
2. Every night, prepare your take-away mid-day meal and refrigerate.
3. Upon rising – greet the day with ½ freshly squeezed lemon juice in 8 oz. filtered water.
4. Prepare Smoothie: Either drink it before you go – or take it with you.
5. If you have time to eat a meal before leaving for the day, eat. This too needs to be well thought out ahead of time.
6. Grab your prepared mid-day meal and hit the road!
7. Supper is planned:
   a) Instant-Pot meal when you get home.
   b) Crockpot meal cooking while you are away.
   c) Left-overs.
   d) Simple ingredients you can throw together without a fuss.

Create an Arsenal of 'Go-to' Meals

Stock your pantry and fridge with ingredients you know how to transform into meals without a lot of bother or mental stress. Favorite go-to meals are a must to keep you sane and on the right track to achieving your health goals.

The salads and entrée's included in this book will become some of your favorites. With pre-planning and the right travel containers you can execute a sustainable, enjoyable and healthy life-style even working full time.

➤ **Take-Away Salad Tips**:

<u>Green Leafy Salads</u>: Keep salad dressing separate in an air-tight sealed container and pour onto salad just before eating.

<u>Bean & Vegetable Salads:</u> Salads with no lettuce can be 'dressed' the night before and 'marinate' in yummy dressing until it's time to eat.

<u>Mock Tuna Chickpea Salad</u>: This salad travels particularly well. Pack chickpea filling separate from long, intact Romaine lettuce leaves and use leaves to scoop up chickpea salad when it's time to eat. Organic brown-rice cakes work well too.

➤ **Take-Away Hot Meal Tips**: *(Remember no microwaves)*.
<u>Purchase a good insulated thermos or wide-mouth container</u>: Pour boiling water into the container to heat thoroughly before adding food. Heat the meal you are taking with you to *hot* and add it to pre-heated container. A thermal insulated container helps retain temperature until meal time.

➤ **Take-Away Cold Meal Tips**:
<u>Ideally, your cold & hot food container will be one & the same</u>. It is important to find the right containers for both hot and cold meals.

Prepare the container to carry cold food by pouring in ice cubes and water, let sit several minutes. Dry and add cold pasta or salad ingredients.

CREATE AN EDD SEVEN-DAY MEAL PLAN

For ultimate detox benefits eat three meals a day – no snacks. Eat to satisfaction, enough to carry you to the next meal. Add Beet & Green Apple Salad once a day to any meal page 180. Plus – drink a Heavy-Metal detox juice once a day, see page 133 for recipe combinations.

Drink smoothies 20 – 30 minutes before eating meal entrée's. Smoothie's are not considered 'meals' but rather healthy, detoxing enhancers to the EDD protocol.

The key to navigating this 21-Day EDD is to plan all the week's meals in advance. Make sure you have all the necessary ingredients for the recipes you've chosen.

Adopt a "Cook Once – Eat Twice" mentality. Soups and stews for dinner and salads for lunch works well. **The EDD Sample Meal Plan** on page 174, is easily adaptable for a busy work schedule.

It is helpful to plan meals and cook a couple meal entrées over the weekend to lessen meal-prep stress during the week. When preparing your evening meal keep in mind what you will take to work for lunch; either save some of the hot entrée or prepare a hearty salad large enough to separate into several lunch portions.

<u>21 Days = 3 weeks.</u> <u>Plan each week's meals in advance.</u>

Each Week:

Include lots of leafy greens, fruits and vegetables. Plan EDD meals around smoothies, salads and delicious, satisfying hot entrées.

1) Choose week's menu & shop for all ingredients.

2) Adopt a cook once – eat twice life-style so each week choose:

   i. <u>2 – 3 Breakfast Entrees' for the work week.</u> Keep it simple like preparing *Over-night Oatmeal; pg 185.* Make a batch of *Pumpkin Pie Rice Pudding; page 188* and *Rice Cream Dream; page 187* to eat throughout the work week.

Choose fun breakfast meals for the weekend like **Sweet Potato Country Hash**, topped with **Roasted Tomatillo Salsa** or **UPMA** Traditional Indian breakfast.

ii. <u>2 – 3 Hearty Salads</u> for cold lunches during the week. **Oil-Free Hummus** is delicious and satisfying, take some along with a salad and a couple organic brown rice cakes for a satisfying mid-day meal that will stave off hunger to dinner.

iii. <u>4 Hot Meal Entrées</u> for evening meals. Separate entrée in half and save second portion for another meal during the week.

7 - DAY EDD SAMPLE MEAL PLAN

Select daily smoothie option & Heavy-Metal Detox Smoothie and purchase all necessary ingredients for the weeks recipes.

Add Beet & Green Apple Salad page180 to one meal each day of the week.

Include a large green leafy salad & oil-free dressing with evening meals.

Three Mid-Week Breakfast = 5 meals:

1. Pumpkin Pie Rice Pudding (x 2) page 188.
2. Rice Cream Dream page (x 2) page 187.
3. Overnight Oatmeal page 185.

Two Fun Weekend Breakfast Entrees:

1. Sweet Potato Country Hash & Roasted Tomatillo Salsa pages 199.
2. UPMA Traditional Indian Breakfast page191.

Three Salad Entrée's = 5 Mid-day Meals:

1. RAW Master Salad & Oil-Free Salad Dressing pages 135.
2. Mock Tuna Salad Chickpea Wraps (x 2) page 195.
3. Mexican Veggie Bean Salad (x 2) page 197.

These salad recipes can be made up ahead of time and stored in lunch portions in the fridge to grab on the way out the door.

Four Hot Entrée Selections = 8 Evening Meals:

1. Louisiana Style Red Beans & Rice (x 2) page 220.
2. Mushroom Lentil Bourguignon & Tasty Mashed Potatoes (x 2) pages 223.
3. Thai Veggie Sauté over Quinoa Pilaf (x 2) pages 219, 215.
4. Old-Fashioned Split-Pea & Potato Soup (x 2) page 209.

Day One:

Upon Rising – drink ½ freshly squeezed lemon in 8 oz. filtered pure water.

Breakfast: Power Punch Green Smoothie
                      Pumpkin Pie Rice Pudding

Mid-Day Meal: RAW Master Salad & Oil-Free Salad Dressing
                      Beet & Green Apple Salad

Supper: Heavy-Metal Detox Smoothie
                      Louisiana Style Red Beans & Rice
                      Large leafy green salad & oil-free dressing

Day Two:

Upon Rising – drink ½ freshly squeezed lemon in 8 oz. filtered pure water.

Breakfast: Health Blast Smoothie
                      Pumpkin Pie Rice Pudding

Mid-Day Meal: Mock Tuna Chickpea Salad Wraps & Romaine Lettuce
                      Two organic brown-rice cakes
                      Beet & Green Apple Salad

Supper: Heavy Metal Detox Smoothie
                      Mushroom Lentil Bourguignon & Tasty Mashed Potatoes
                      Large green leafy salad & oil free dressing

Day Three:

Upon Rising – drink ½ freshly squeezed lemon add 1 tsp apple-cider vinegar in 8 oz. pure filtered water.

Breakfast: Heavenly Green Smoothie
                  Over-night Oatmeal

Mid-Day Meal: Mock Tuna Chickpea Salad Wraps & Romaine Lettuce
                  2 organic brown rice cakes
                  Beet & Green Apple Salad

Supper: Heavy-Metal Detox Smoothie
                  Thai Veggie Sauté over Quinoa Pilaf
                  Large green leafy salad & oil free dressing

Day Four:

Upon Rising – drink ½ freshly squeezed lemon add 1 tsp apple-cider vinegar in 8 oz. pure filtered water.

Breakfast: Berry Blend Delight
                  Rice Cream Dream

Mid-Day Meal: Mexican Veggie Bean Salad
                  2 organic brown rice cakes
                  Beet & Green Apple Salad

Supper: Heavy-Metal Detox Smoothie
                  Old-Fashioned Split-Pea & Potato Soup
                  Large green leafy salad & oil-free dressing

Day Five:

Upon Rising – drink ½ freshly squeezed lemon add 1 tsp apple-cider vinegar and 1 tsp non-aluminum baking soda in 8 oz. filtered pure water. Mixture will foam up and carbonate a bit. You can work up to 1-Tablespoon vinegar if you can handle it.

Breakfast: Powerhouse Punch Green Smoothie
                        Rice Cream Dream

Mid-Day Meal: Mexican Veggie Bean Salad
                        Beet & Green Apple Salad

Supper: Heavy-Metal Detox Smoothie
                        Louisiana Red Beans & Rice
                        Large green leafy salad & oil-free dressing

Weekend Day Six:

Upon Rising – drink ½ freshly squeezed lemon add 1 tsp apple-cider vinegar and 1 tsp non-aluminum baking soda in 8 oz. filtered pure water. Mixture will foam up and carbonate a bit.

Breakfast: Melon or fruit salad – 20 minutes later;
                        Sweet Potato Country Hash & Roasted Tomatillo Salsa

Mid-Day Meal: Oil-free Hummus, Mango Salsa & Raw Veggie platter plus
                        organic brown rice cakes for dipping

Supper: Heavy-Metal Detox Smoothie
                        Mushroom Lentil Bourguignon & Tasty Mashed Potatoes
                        Large green leafy salad & oil free dressing

Weekend Day Seven:

Upon Rising – drink ½ freshly squeezed lemon add 1 tsp apple-cider vinegar and 1 tsp non-aluminum baking soda in 8 oz. filtered pure water. Mixture will foam up and carbonate a bit.

Breakfast: Health Blast Smoothie page
        UPMA – Traditional Indian Breakfast

Mid-Day Meal: Thai Veggie Sauté over Quinoa Pilaf
        Beet Salad & Green Apple Salad

Supper: Heavy-Metal Detox Smoothie
        Old Fashioned Split-Pea & Potato Soup
        Large leafy green salad & oil free dressing

Chapter 18

ELIMINATION DETOX DIET RECIPES

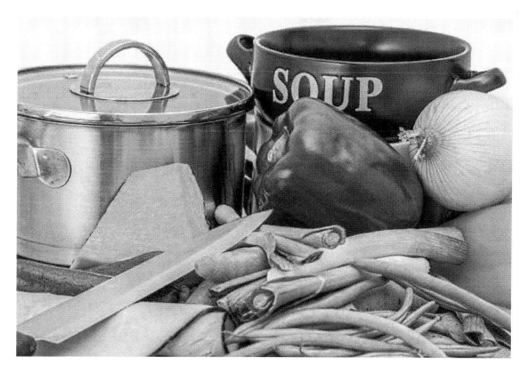

Once a Day – Eat Beets & Green Apples for DETOX

Beets and green apples are particularly cleansing for the blood and colon and stimulates bowel function. It is recommended you consume this *Beet Salad*, or *Apple Beet Salad* once daily with any of your three meals. If you HATE eating beets, try adding a little beet to your juice smoothies and see if you can handle it and work up from there.

Beet Salad Recipe

Yields: 1 serving (depending on beet size)

- 1 medium-sized raw beet, peeled and grated
- Juice of half a lemon *(or more if you prefer)*
- Dijon mustard and fresh ginger root adds flavor and kicks it up a bit.

Apple Beet Salad Option:

- Grate one green apple into above ingredients to make a beet & apple salad. It is surprisingly refreshing!

Be sure to chew raw beets and apples thoroughly.

EDD Breakfast Inspirations

Smoothie Choices:

These recipes are an inspirational launching point – if a fruit is listed here and you don't have it, substitute another and be creative. If you can't eat bananas skip them and add frozen or fresh fruit, it's all good.

BERRY BLEND DELIGHT

Yields: 2 large or 4 small servings

Ingredients:

- 1 - 2 cups frozen unsweetened berry blend; raspberries, strawberries, cherries or blueberries *(Costco carries a frozen organic blend)*
- ¾ cup chilled unsweetened almond or rice milk
- 1 frozen banana *(optional)*
- 1 tsp ground flaxseed
- 2 tsp finely grated fresh ginger
- 2 tsp fresh lemon juice

COMBINE all ingredients in blender, adding lemon juice to taste. Puree until smooth. Pour into 2 chilled glasses.

FROTHY BANANA STRAWBERRY FRUIT SMOOTHIE

Yields: 1 serving

- 1 – 2 frozen bananas
- 4 to 6 frozen organic strawberries
- ½ to 1 cup unfiltered organic apple juice
- 1 tsp vanilla
- Adding a sprig or two of fresh mint adds a delicious flavor – optional.

Directions: Mix in heavy-duty blender and enjoy.

POWERHOUSE PUNCH GREEN SMOOTHIE

Yields: 2 large, or 4 small servings

Ingredients:

- 1 ½ cups filtered water *(with ice if desired)*
- 2 large green apples, peeled, cored and roughly chopped
- 2 cups packed kale and / or spinach
- 2/3 cup loosely packed fresh parsley leaves
- 1/3 cup packed fresh cilantro leaves* and or mint
- 1/2 cup frozen mango chunks, or frozen pineapple, or strawberries or whatever organic fruit you have on hand.
- 1 frozen banana *(optional)*
- ½ avocado
- ½ - 1 fresh squeezed lemon juice
- 2 small pieces fresh turmeric**

Directions:

1. Add the water into a high-speed blender.
2. Now add the rest of the ingredients. Blend on high until super smooth. If you have a Vitamix, use the tamper stick to get things moving.

Serve and enjoy! Place any leftovers into an airtight container and store in the fridge for up to 24 hours.

➤ **Tips:**
- * If you aren't a cilantro fan, feel free to add more kale, spinach or fresh mint.
- ** Fresh turmeric root is anti-inflammatory and is orange in color, small and tubular. It can be found at Sprouts and other health food stores, and Indian and Asian grocery stores. If you can't find it make the juice without it.

HEAVENLY GREEN SMOOTHIE

Yields: 2 large – or 4 small servings

Ingredients:

- 1 orange, peeled
- 1 cup seedless, stemmed grapes *(frozen works great!)*
- 1 banana *(frozen works great!)*
- 1 green apple; peeled & cored
- 1 cup unsweetened coconut, almond, or rice milk
- 2 cups fresh kale or spinach

Place all ingredients in a high-power blender for 1 minute, or until desired smoothness is achieved.

HEALTH BLAST JUICE!

Yields: 2 large – or 4 small servings

This is not the tasty berry & banana fruit smoothie. No, this one packs a powerful punch – and can be a little 'hot' depending on the jalapeno & ginger. This is a particularly healing, alkalizing and detoxing recipe.

If you are combating a cancer diagnosis, or recovering from chemo, or desire to kick up detox benefits – this juice is a great way to optimize the healing process.

- 1/2 medium red beet – or one whole small beet
- 3 stalks kale
- 3 celery stalks
- 1/4 bunch cilantro
- 1/4 bunch parsley
- 2 green apples
- 1 lemon – peeled
- 1 orange – peeled
- 3 inches ginger root
- 3 inches turmeric root
- 1/4 jalapeno – seeded

Directions – add all ingredients to your *juicer* – NOT the blender – unless you strain it. There is too much pulp in this juice to merely blend and try to gag down. Enjoy the healthy blast!

OVERNIGHT BREAKFAST OATS

Oats are naturally gluten-free; but if you are Celiac read the package carefully to verify oats are prepared in a dedicated gluten-free facility.

Preparing overnight oats is a wonderful way to greet the morning – or a convenient, nutritious breakfast to take with you on the go!

There are creative flavor profiles for over-night oatmeal. Below the basic oatmeal recipe are several flavor profile options. Build the basic recipe, then add additional fruits & spices for variety.

Yields: 1 serving. You will need an air-tight sealing glass jar.

Basic Ingredients:

- 1/3 cup plain non-dairy organic yogurt- *NOT soy base*
- ½ cup (*heaping*) rolled oats
- 2/3 cup unsweetened non-dairy milk; coconut, almond, rice, hemp
- 1 Tbsp. chia seeds or ground flax meal
- ½ tsp pure vanilla extract
- Pinch of salt
- 1 – 2 tsp raw honey or pure maple syrup

Option: Old Fashioned Overnight Oatmeal:

- 1 tsp cinnamon
- ½ tsp nutmeg
- ¼ tsp cloves
- ¼ tsp allspice
- ¼ cup raisins

Add other flavors & ingredients as desired; see suggestions below.

Directions:

1. Whisk all ingredients together in a medium-sized bowl. Spoon into an air-tight glass container with tight-fitting lid. Refrigerate for a minimum of 4 hours, but overnight is preferred.

Overnight Oatmeal Flavor Options:

Carrot Cake: To the list of Old Fashioned Oatmeal ingredients above, add 1 small peeled, grated carrot.

Banana Strawberry: Use basic recipe and add 1 chopped banana, and several chopped fresh strawberries.

Tropical Fruit: Use basic recipe and add chopped mangos, and / or pineapple, ¼ cup unsweetened flaked coconut.

RAW Apple Compote

Yields: 1 – 2 servings

This tart applesauce makes a great extra detoxing side dish to accompany a breakfast porridge OR mid-day salad, soup, or stew.

Ingredients:

- 2 tart apples, cored & diced
- 1 – 2 tsp ginger, freshly grated (*or ½ tsp dried*)
- ½ tsp cinnamon, powdered
- ¼ cup parsley, fresh, stems removed, or fresh mint chopped fine

Directions:

1. Blend apples, ginger, cinnamon, and fresh parsley. If you are mixing this by hand, grate the apple first and finely chop the parsley.

The parsley tastes surprisingly divine in apple sauce. Start with a small amount if you aren't sure. You can even go up to a whole cup – or more if desired.

HOT CEREAL – PORRIGE SELECTIONS

RICE CREAM DREAM

Yields: 2 – 3 servings

Ingredients:

- ½ cup long grain rice, uncooked
- 2 cups water
- ½ tsp salt
- ½ tsp cinnamon, powdered
- ¼ tsp cardamom, powdered
- ¼ cup unsweetened non-dairy milk; *coconut, almond or rice*
- 1 Tbsp. flax seeds *(or seed of choice)*

Directions:

1. In a medium saucepan, combine rice, water, salt, cinnamon, and cardamom.
2. Bring to a boil. Cover. Reduce heat. Simmer for 20 minutes, or until tender. Remove from heat, keep covered, and let it sit for 5 minutes before serving.
3. For a creamy consistency, puree in a blender or food processor with non-dairy milk.
4. Optional: garnish with seed of choice.

PUMPKIN PIE RICE PUDDING

This is surprisingly delicious and reminiscent of pumpkin pie. A real treat. You'll feel like you are cheating with this one!

Yields: 2 – 3 servings

After the EDD, add chopped pecans and maple syrup and it tastes like a bowl of pumpkin pie comfort food! *BUT,* it's healthy!

Ingredients:

- 1 cup basmati rice, uncooked; rinse and drain *(or any long grain rice)*
- 3 cups water or unsweetened rice milk
- 1 cup pumpkin, peeled and cubed; or canned, organic *(or sweet potato or winter squash)*
- 1 tsp cinnamon
- 1 tsp ginger, freshly grated *(or ½ tsp powdered ginger)*
- ¼ tsp cloves, ground *(or 3 whole cloves; removed after cooking)*
- ¼ tsp nutmeg
- ½ tsp salt

Directions:

1. Combine all ingredients in a medium saucepan.
2. Cover. Bring to a boil. Reduce heat and simmer for 20 – 45 minutes, or until rice and pumpkin are soft. Remove from heat and let sit for 5 minutes covered before serving. Puree or mash together for a creamy consistency.

GINGER MILLET SKILLET

Yields: 1 – 2 servings

Ingredients:

- 1 cup millet, soaked, drained and dried with a tea towel or paper towels *(or organic gluten-free grain blend, or grain of your choice)*
- 3 cups water
- 2 tsp ginger, fresh, grated *(or 1 tsp powdered ginger)*
- ½ tsp cinnamon, ground
- ¼ tsp cloves, ground *(or 3 whole cloves; removed before serving)*
- ¼ tsp salt
- 1 Tbsp. flax seeds (or seed of your choice), whole

Spice amounts are a suggestions; season to your personal taste.

Directions:

1. In a large dry saucepan, toast the millet at medium heat for 3 – 5 minutes, until it smells nutty, stirring constantly.
2. Add the water, ginger, cinnamon, cloves and salt to the pan.
3. Cover. Bring to a boil. Reduce heat to low. Simmer for 15 minutes.
4. Remove from heat and let sit covered for 10 minutes before serving.
5. Garnish with flax, chia, hemp or sesame seeds.

SWEET POTATO COUNTRY HASH

Yields: 2 servings

Ingredients:

- 2 large sweet potatoes or yams peeled & chopped *(you can use any potatoes for this recipe; peel russet potatoes, but no need to peel yellow or red potatoes. If using smaller potatoes, use 4-6 small potatoes for two servings, or 2-3 for one serving)*
- ½ cup vegetable broth or water to sauté *(approximate; add as needed)*
- ½ yellow, orange or red bell pepper
- 4-5 green onions; chopped *(or ½ chopped small onion of your choice; purple, sweet, white, brown)*
- 2 heaping tsps minced garlic
- ½ cup chopped fresh parsley *(or, 2 Tbsp. dried)*
- ½ cup chopped spinach *(or more if you prefer, spinach reduces when cooked)*
- 1 cup mushrooms; chopped *(optional, but adds cancer-fighting nutrients and chewy, satisfaction)*
- Salt & pepper to taste
- Herbs are fun here – use your imagination and add your favorites; tarragon, basil, cilantro, rosemary, thyme

Directions:

1. Sauté onions and bell pepper in 2-3 Tbsp. of vegetable broth or water until soft and translucent, about 2-3 minutes.
2. Add garlic, and stir until fragrant.
3. Add potatoes and stir to mix well. You will need more vegetable broth here, keep an eye on the potatoes, and add broth sparingly so potatoes do not burn.
4. Cover and cook potatoes until *almost* tender.
5. Add parsley, spinach and mushrooms, stir to mix and cook until potatoes are tender. *Top with avocado and salsa if desired.*

UPMA (Traditional Indian Breakfast)

Yields: 1 – 2 servings

Ingredients:

- ½ cup brown rice, uncooked *(grind rice in a Ninja or a coffee grinder until cereal consistency – not powder)*
- 2 cups water
- ½ cup carrot, chopped
- ½ cup peas *(we use frozen petite peas)*
- 1 cup green beans, chopped (*organic frozen green beans are sold at Costco and other health conscious grocery stores)*
- 1 ½ tsp cumin seeds
- ¼ tsp ground black pepper
- ½ tsp salt

Directions:

1. Toast the cumin seeds *(optional, but the smell and flavor is divine!).* Heat a heavy skillet over medium heat. Add the cumin seeds and toast 2 – 5 minutes or until fragrant and lightly browned, stirring constantly to prevent burning. Remove from heat.
2. Add ¼ cup water, carrots, peas, green beans, salt & pepper. Water sauté over medium heat until tender.
3. Meanwhile, in a small saucepan, add brown rice cereal, 1 ¾ cups of water, and a pinch of salt. Bring to a boil while stirring. Reduce heat to low. Cover and simmer for 5 – 8 minutes until creamy. Remove from heat and stir until smooth.
4. Combine the cooked rice cereal with the vegetables and serve.

EDD Salad Entrée Selections

Salads & Oil Free Dressing Recipes

Included here are several salad and oil-free salad dressing recipes. You can search online for *"vegan, oil-free, soy-free salad dressings"* for a gazillion creative ideas that work well with the EDD. Find your favorites, mix them up in quadruple batches and keep them in an air-tight jar in the fridge for convenience.

RAW 'MASTER' VEGETABLE SALAD – Page 135

In the *How to Detox* Chapter, there is a list of ingredients for the RAW 'MASTER' Salad and salad dressing. This salad mixture is a wonderful way to detox your body while enjoying a delicious, crunchy fresh salad.

Build yourself the RAW MASTER SALAD – and use any one of these oil-free dressings for a delicious, nutritious, detoxing salad.

OIL - FREE SALAD DRESSING RECIPES

Fat-Free Cilantro Zucchini Dressing

Yields: 3-4 servings

- 1 zucchini, chopped
- ½ cup lime or lemon juice
- ¼ - ½ cup cilantro, freshly chopped
- ¼ cup water
- ½ tsp salt
- ¼ tsp black pepper, freshly ground

Directions: Blend all ingredients in a blender or food processor until smooth.

Sweet Tangy Thai Dressing:

- ½ fresh squeezed lime – or more if desired
- 1 Tbsp. sweet chili sauce (*watch sugar content on this*)
- 1 Tbsp. rice vinegar
- 1 Tbsp. Liquid Aminos – *or low sodium organic soy sauce*
- 2 Tbsp. cold filtered water
- 2 Tbsp. cilantro, chopped – or mint
- 1 tsp garlic, minced
- 1 tsp ginger, minced
- 1 tsp raw honey

Directions: Mix up this dressing and taste & season according to your preference before pouring on your salad.

Option: If you like spicy hot – sprinkle with red chili flakes, or add oriental ground chili paste to taste.

Oil-Free Creamy Vinaigrette

Ingredients:

- 3 Tbsp. plain unsweetened non-dairy (*not soy based*) yogurt
- 3 Tbsp. fresh squeezed orange juice
- 3 Tbsp. chopped fresh cilantro or parsley
- 2 Tbsp. water
- 2 Tbsp. white wine vinegar
- 2 Tbsp. lime juice
- 1 tsp chili powder
- 1/2 tsp onion powder
- 1/2 tsp ground cumin

Directions: Combine all ingredients in a covered jar. Shake to mix. Use at once or refrigerate for later use.

<u>Oil-Free Vegan Ranch Dressing</u>

Ingredients:

- 3 Tbsp. plain, unsweetened non-dairy *(not soy)* yogurt
- 2 Tbsp. water
- 2 Tbsp. fresh squeeze lemon juice
- 1 Tbsp. dry parsley
- 1 Tbsp. dried dill
- 1 tsp granulated onion
- ½ tsp salt
- ½ tsp raw honey
- ¼ tsp granulated garlic

Directions: Crush dry herbs in palm of hand as you add to mixing bowl. Mix all ingredients and serve. Saves well in airtight container.

> Tip: Mix up a triple recipe and store in jar in fridge for next time.

<u>Oil-Free Balsamic Vinaigrette</u>

Yields: 1/4 cup

Ingredients:

- 2 Tbsp. balsamic vinegar
- 2 Tbsp. seasoned rice vinegar
- 1 Tbsp. *organic* ketchup
- 1 tsp stone-ground mustard
- 1 tsp minced garlic or fresh clove

Raspberry Vinaigrette Option:

- Substitute raspberry vinegar for balsamic vinegar and omit garlic in your salad for a fun alternative.

Directions: Whisk vinegars, ketchup, mustard, and garlic together. Taste and season according to your preference.

'MOCK TUNA' CHICKPEA SALAD WRAPS

Yields: Approximately 4 large wraps

In this recipe, salad becomes finger food and tuna is replaced with chickpeas as leaves of romaine lettuce are used to wrap a tasty chickpea filling.

This makes a refreshing wrap that's high in healthful fiber. This chickpea mixture is a great substitute for tuna in a sandwich.

Ingredients:

- 1 ½ cups cooked or canned chickpeas, rinsed and drained
- ¼ cup toasted sunflower seeds (*optional but they add a great crunch!*)
- ½ cup finely chopped or grated carrot
- ½ cup finely chopped celery
- ¼ cup chopped cilantro, parsley or mint
- 3 green onions, chopped (*you can substitute purple onion or even add both*)
- 1 – 2 Tbsp. stone-ground mustard
- 1 Tbsp. rice wine vinegar or vinegar of your choice
- ½ tsp pink salt
- ¼ tsp ground black pepper – or fresh ground pepper to taste
- 1 tsp raw organic honey
- 4 large romaine lettuce leaves
- 1 medium tomato, sliced, or 6 to 8 cherry tomatoes, cut in half

Directions:

1. Coarsely mash the beans with a fork or potato masher, leaving some chunks. Add the remaining ingredients. Mix well & season to taste.
2. Place about one-quarter of the mixture on each lettuce leaf. Add one-quarter of the tomato, roll the lettuce around the filling, and serve.
3. Store in a covered container in the refrigerator. Leftover Chickpea Salad (*without the lettuce and tomato*) will keep for up to 3 days.

CRUNCHY BROCCOLI SALAD

This salad is best chilled for a minimum of 2 hours – and even overnight if you have the time. It saves very well in an airtight container for up to five days in the refrigerator.

Yields: approximately 5 cups.

Ingredients:

- 4 cups broccoli florets – cut into bite size pieces
- ¼ cup raw – or toasted sunflower seeds or toasted almond slivers
- ½ cup raisins
- ½ cup purple onions, diced
- 1 peeled & grated carrot
- *Optional; cherry tomatoes cut in 1/2, or diced fresh tomatoes.*

Directions:

1. Pour boiling water over raisins and soak to plump while you prepare other ingredients; 5 – 10 minutes. Don't worry you can't over plump! Drain thoroughly.
2. Toast sunflower seeds in non-stick pan until they are toasty and brown. Shake often and watch carefully so they don't burn.
3. In medium mixing bowl add broccoli, chopped onions, carrot, and toasted sunflower seeds.
4. Drain raisins & add to broccoli mixture.
5. Add dressing to broccoli salad – and enjoy!

Chill for up to two hours for a richer flavor. This salad can be eaten cold or at room temperature.

> *Tip:* Try variations of salad dressings to suit your taste profile – see Oil-Free Dressing recipe selections on pages 192-194.

MEXICAN VEGGIE & BEAN SALAD

Yields: 6-8 servings

Ingredients:

- 1 15-ounce can organic garbanzo or cannellini beans
- 1 15-ounce can organic kidney beans
- 1 15-ounce can organic black beans
- 1 large cucumber, peeled and diced
- ½ cup finely chopped red onion
- 1 medium red bell pepper, seeded and finely diced
- 1 medium tomato, seeded and diced
- ½ cup chopped fresh cilantro
- 2 Tbsp. seasoned rice vinegar
- 2 Tbsp. apple cider vinegar or distilled vinegar
- 1 Tbsp. lemon or lime juice
- 1 garlic clove, minced
- 1 tsp ground cumin
- 1 tsp ground coriander
- 1/8 tsp cayenne pepper

Optional: Top with chunks of avocado

Directions:

1. In a large salad bowl, combine, cucumber, onion, bell pepper, tomato, and cilantro.
2. In a small bowl, combine vinegars, lemon or lime juice, garlic, cumin, coriander, and cayenne. Pour over the salad and toss gently to mix. Salad tastes best when chilled at least one hour before serving. Also, can be made and refrigerated overnight.

MEDITERRANEAN STYLE SPROUTED QUINOA SALAD

Yields: 8 – 10 *servings*

This is the PERFECT salad to take with you to work, to potlucks, and to social food gatherings where "health-conscious" food choices may be scarce. Your friends and co-workers are going to love this one!

You can use all quinoa – or a quinoa rice blend. TruRoots sells wonderful products – check them out at: http://www.truroots.com/products/truroots-accents/organic-accents-sprouted-quinoa-trio.

Ingredients:

- 2 cups dry quinoa or quinoa rice blend – cook according to package directions; should yield four cups when cooked
- 1 - 2 grated carrots; depending on how large they are
- ¾ cup chopped basil, cilantro, and/or parsley
- 1 small grated or chopped zucchini
- ¼ cup diced purple onion *(green onion works well here too)*
- ½ - ¾ cup diced yellow or red bell pepper
- 1 cup sliced black olives
- 1 small diced tomato
- 1 cup chopped fresh spinach - or kale - your preference
- 1 can drained & rinsed red kidney beans *(black beans are also delicious)*

Directions

1. Cook quinoa blend according to package directions. Be careful not to overcook, salad is best when quinoa rice blend is slightly chewy.
2. Chop vegetables while quinoa cooks.
3. Mix quinoa blend, vegetables and beans together.
4. Top with your favorite *oil-free* dressing & mix well to coat all ingredients.
5. Refrigerate until serving.

Salad stays good in the refrigerate for 3 – 4 days.

ROASTED TOMATILLO – SALSA VERDE

This outstanding green salsa can be poured hot over roasted root vegetables; mashed potatoes, rice or breakfast country style potatoes. It can be added to soups and stews and added cold to spice up the Mexican Vegetable Salad. It's a great dip with rice cakes and hummus. Experiment and enjoy!

Yields: About 2 - 3 cups

Ingredients:

- 1 pound fresh tomatillos
- 3 fresh serrano chilies, or green chilies, split open and seeded
- 2 poblano chilies, split in two and seeded
- 1 whole garlic clove; separate cloves, but do not peel
- 1 large onion, roughly chopped
- Salt and freshly ground black pepper
- ½ cup fresh cilantro leaves; chopped
- ¼ cup vegetable broth, or more as needed

Directions:

1. Preheat broiler to high – about 550 F
2. Lightly spray a cookie sheet with scant amount of coconut nonstick spray.
3. Remove husks from the tomatillos and rinse under warm water to remove stickiness. Cut tomatillos in half and place face side down on prepared cookie sheet. Place split open and flattened chilies face side down on pan – add garlic cloves and chopped onion. Drizzle with small amount of vegetable broth; just enough to barely dampen vegetables & sprinkle with salt & fresh ground pepper.
4. Place on upper rack in broiler about 1 – 2 inches from heat and cook, turning the vegetables once, until softened and slightly charred, about 5 to 7 minutes. When garlic cloves are cool enough to handle, peel skin. I find holding it by one end and squeezing it like a toothpaste tube works well.
5. Add all the broiled ingredients to a blender along with the fresh cilantro. Pour in ¼ cup vegetable broth and blend to puree. Add more broth if needed for desired consistency.

VEGAN TACO SALAD

We use <u>TruRoots Sprouted Quinoa or TruRoots Brown Rice Blend</u> for the filling of this tasty Vegan Taco Salad; see recipe on page 202, for TruRoots info.

Make this delicious 'taco' filling and use it as a base and top with your favorite taco salad ingredients.

Suggested Taco Salad Ingredients: Tomato, romaine & red leafy lettuce, fresh chopped spinach, purple onions, cilantro, sliced or chopped avocados, mango salsa *(recipe page 198)* or add your favorite taco sauce.

Yields: 4 - 6 Taco Salad Servings

Filling Ingredients:

- 1 cup (dry measure) Sprouted Rice or Quinoa Blend. Cook *'al dente'* according to package directions
- ¼ cup veggie broth for sautéing
- 1 15 oz. can organic tomato sauce
- 1 4 oz. can diced green chilies *(Or 1 fresh green chili, seeded & chopped)*
- 1 cup sliced black olives
- 1 medium purple onion diced
- 2 heaping tsp crushed garlic
- 1 - 2 Tbsp. of chili powder *(Season to taste)*
- 1 - 2 tsp cumin powder
- 1 tsp dried oregano
- 1 tsp smoked or sweet paprika
- ½ cup chopped fresh parsley
- ½ cup chopped fresh cilantro
- 1 tsp pink Himalayan, Kosher or sea salt
- Cracked black pepper to taste
- Pepitas, or toasted pumpkin seeds go well on this salad. Or, top with raw or toasted sunflower seeds.

Directions:

1. Cook 1 cup sprouted rice & quinoa blend; or favorite organic wild rice blend according to package directions. - *Do not overcook* - you want texture to be chewy - almost al dente. Keep a watch on the fluid levels, sometimes you need to add a little more water toward the end of cooking time.
2. When rice / quinoa blend is cooked to a nice chewy 'al dente' remove from heat and set aside.
3. It is a good idea to prep and chop all taco filling ingredients while the rice / quinoa blend is cooking.
4. In a large non-stick skillet sauté the purple onion and garlic in ¼ cup veggie broth. If using a fresh green chili, add it now and cook until vegetables are softened and translucent.
5. If using canned green chilies add now along with all remaining filling ingredients; black olives, tomato sauce & spices, parsley & cilantro.
6. Taste & season to your preference.
7. Once tomato - vegetable mixture is bubbly hot and seasoned to your liking, add the al dente cooked rice / quinoa blend. You do not want the taco filling to continue to "cook" and become mushy, mix until well blended, hot and a nice chewy consistency then remove from heat.
8. Build Taco Salad & and *enjoy!* You can place mixture in the middle of a dinner plate and top with fresh taco salad toppings. Or, load your plate with your favorite fresh taco salad ingredients and scoop the hot taco filling over the top.

> **Tip: VEGAN TACOS** - *After EDD* – use this filling to create vegan tacos. Use only *organic* - non-GMO Verified corn tortillas, and *organic* non-GMO verified Canola oil to cook taco shells.

MANGO SALSA

This delicious salsa can be served hot; scooped over Mexican Butternut Squash, or Mexican Lentil Chili, or Vegan Taco Salad. Or cold, served up on a nice salad plate along with Oil-Free Hummus, Crunchy Broccoli Salad, or a fresh crisp spinach salad.

Ingredients:

- ¼ cup vegetable broth
- 1 large onion, diced
- 1 ½ tsp fresh minced garlic
- 1 Tbsp. fresh minced ginger
- 1 small jalapeno seeded, or 1 fresh green chili, seeded and chopped, or one small 4 oz. can of mild green chilis *(See Tip below)*
- ¼ cup minced cilantro – or fresh mint
- 2 ripe mangos chopped – or 2 – 3 cups frozen, defrosted mango. Or, if your local grocer sells canned mangos, use one – two cans, drained and chopped
- ½ cup freshly squeezed orange juice. Or, peel a fresh orange and thoroughly liquefy it in a food processor or high-powered blender; this adds delicious bulk to salsa
- 1 tsp sea salt, pink or Kosher salt
- Fresh cracked black pepper to taste
- Optional; 1 tsp raw honey – adjust depending on sweetness of mango
- Optional; Add a couple drops smoky chipotle hot sauce

➢ **Tip:** The longer you cook the jalapeno, the hotter the salsa will become. If you like it hot – add the jalapeno when you add the onion. If you like it REAL HOT add the seeds. If you don't like hot – be careful here; use a smaller portion of jalapeno, or only cook long enough to soften the jalapeno.

➢ If you like a very mild, flavorful salsa – skip the jalapeno and add 1 small can diced green chilies. Or substitute the jalapeno for one large green chili, seeded and chopped and proceed with above directions.

Directions:

1. Sauté onions broth until translucent, about 10 minutes.
2. Add garlic and ginger and cook until fragrance is released.
3. Add jalapeno and cook until soft.
4. Add cilantro, or mint and stir to mix well.
5. Add mango, orange juice, honey (*if using*), salt and pepper.
6. Cook until well combined. Taste and adjust seasonings.
7. Salsa can be served warm, at room temperature, or chilled.

DELICIOUS OIL-FREE HUMMUS!

Yields: approximately 3 cups prepared

Ingredients:

- Two 15 oz. cans organic garbanzo beans; RESERVE liquid in separate bowl; rinse and drain beans
- ¼ - ½ cup reserved garbanzo bean liquid
- Approximately ½ - ¾ cup fresh lemon juice; juice of 2 to 4 lemons – according to your own taste.
- ½ cup tahini (*sesame seed butter; looks like peanut butter*)
- 3 Tbsp. cumin; or more (*season according to taste*)
- Loads of fresh minced garlic; approx. 2 tablespoons – or more according to your taste
- Approximately 1 ½ tsp Kosher, Pink Himalayan or sea salt
- ½ tsp black pepper (flavor to taste)

Optional: Sprinkle lightly with paprika.

> Tip: **AFTER EDD** – drizzle a small amount of organic extra-virgin olive oil on top.

Directions

1. Add garbanzo beans, ½ cup lemon juice, garlic, tahini, ¼ cup reserved garbanzo bean liquid and salt & pepper to food processor and process until smooth.
2. Add more reserved liquid if necessary for a smooth, spreadable consistency.
3. Taste and adjust lemon juice, garlic, cumin, salt & pepper to your preference.

> Tip: Hummus is packed with healthy protein. Add a scoop to your favorite salad – or chop a slew of your favorite veggies and dip away!

SAVORY EDD SOUP ENTRÉE SELECTIONS

VEGETABLE MINESTRONE SOUP

Yields: 6 – 8 servings

Use organic canned beans – or soak an assortment of dry beans overnight and cook the beans 1 – 2 hours or until tender and then follow directions below.

Ingredients:

- 1 can kidney beans
- 1 can white navy beans – or cannellini
- 1 can black beans
- 1 onion, peeled and chopped
- 2 carrots, peeled and copped
- 2 stalks celery, peel outer strings
- 2 – 3 heaping tsp minced garlic – *according to taste*
- 1 28-ounce can crushed tomatoes *(more if you love tomatoes)*
- 3 medium potatoes chopped into bite size portions
- ½ cup loosely packed parsley leaves, chopped
- 2 – 4 Tbsp. chopped fresh basil; according to your taste
- 3 Tbsp. fresh chopped oregano, or 2 Tbsp. dry
- *(Optional)* ½ chopped fennel
- Salt & pepper to taste

Directions:

1. Rinse and drain beans if using canned. Soak and cook beans if using dry.
2. In a large Dutch oven or soup pot, sauté chopped onions in small amount of veggie broth until translucent. Add garlic and cook until fragrant.
3. Stir in *all* remaining ingredients and cover vegetables with clean filtered water or vegetable broth until it is covered by 1 inch.
4. Raise the heat and bring to a boil. Reduce heat and simmer uncovered until vegetables are tender and ready to eat.

➤ **Tip: After EDD** – *add pasta such as Israeli couscous or organic pasta shells. Cook the pasta according to package directions until it is al dente (slightly chewy) and then add pasta to the fully cooked soup.*

CREAM OF ASPARAGUS HERB SOUP

Yields: approximately 4 servings

Ingredients:

- 2 bunches asparagus, trim bottom 2-inches, slightly peel outside layer for less strings in finished soup. Dice into *small* pieces
- 1 large onion, white sweet onions have a lot of flavor
- 1 – 2 tsp minced garlic
- 4 – 5 cups low-sodium vegetable broth
- 1 large peeled carrot finely diced
- 1 ½ tsp pink Himalayan salt, Kosher salt, or sea salt *(to taste)*
- ¼ cup fresh minced thyme – or 2 tsp dried
- ¼ cup fresh minced tarragon – or 2 – 3 tsp dried
- Fresh black pepper to taste

This soup lends itself well to a variety of seasonings; Indian, Italian and Mexican see season chart.

Directions:

1. Sauté diced onion in small amount of veggie broth.
2. When onions are translucent add garlic and diced carrots, cook and stir. another 5 minutes or so.
3. Add asparagus, salt, pepper, seasons and herbs, mix well.
4. Add vegetable stock & bring to a boil.
5. Reduce heat and cook approximately 30 minutes, or until soft.
6. Give one last taste and season accordingly.
7. Use immersion blender to mix into a creamy soup. OR – carefully pour hot mixture into a heavy-duty blender and blend until *very* smooth. An immersion blender may not adequately pulverize strings, as asparagus tends to be stringy, so be sure to blend well for a smooth, satisfying creamy soup.

CREAMY CHEESY BROCCOLI SOUP

Yields: approximately 4 servings

Ingredients:

- 4 cups trimmed broccoli florets
- 1 large onion, white sweet onions have a lot of flavor
- 1 – 2 tsp minced garlic
- 4 – 5 cups low-sodium vegetable broth
- 2-3 large peeled carrots finely diced
- 1 ½ tsp pink Himalayan salt, Kosher salt, or sea salt *(to taste)*
- ¼ cup fresh minced thyme – or 2 tsp dried
- ¼ cup fresh minced tarragon – or 2 – 3 tsp dried
- 2 Tbsp. Nutritional Yeast
- Fresh black pepper to taste

This soup lends itself well to a variety of seasonings; Indian, Italian and Mexican see season chart.

Directions:

1. Sauté diced onion in small amount of veggie broth.
2. When onions are translucent add garlic and diced carrots, cook and stir. another 5 minutes or so.
3. Add broccoli, salt, pepper, seasons and herbs, mix well.
4. Add vegetable stock & bring to a boil.
5. Reduce heat and cook approximately 30 minutes, or until soft.
6. Give one last taste and season accordingly.
7. Carefully pour hot mixture into a heavy-duty blender and blend until *very* smooth.
8. Add Nutritional Yeast – and blend briefly to thoroughly mix, but do not *over blend* as NY tends to make soups 'gelatinous' when over blended.

If you desire a more vegetable rich mouthful experience, feel free to NOT 'cream' the soup in the blender.

SWEET SPICY THAI NOODLE SOUP

Yields: 2 – 4 servings

What a delicious way to enjoy healthy green vegetables! Feel free to spice this one up according to your flavor profile – hot & spicy or mild.

Ingredients:

- 1 Tbsp. finely minced fresh ginger or, *you can find jarred minced ginger in produce section of local grocery store*
- 1 Tbsp. minced garlic
- ½ - 1 jalapeño pepper, seeded and finely chopped
- 6 cups vegetable broth; *more or less depending thickness you prefer*
- 3 – 4 Tbsp. low-sodium organic soy sauce; or Liquid Aminos
- ½ - 1 tsp Chinese garlic chili sauce; *to taste*
- 3 Tbsp. sherry
- 1 Tbsp. mirin
- 1 Tbsp. Better than Vegetable Bouillon
- 2 tsp smoked sesame seed oil
- 2 cups sliced mushrooms
- 1 peeled, grated carrot
- 1 cup bite-size broccoli florets
- 1 cup packed finely chopped bok choy
- 1 cup fresh packed spinach, diced (*optional*)
- 2 – 3 green onions, finely chopped, including top
- ¼ cup finely chopped fresh cilantro
- 1 cup *cooked* Asian rice noodles; or 100% buckwheat soba noodles

Directions:

1. Sauté ginger, garlic, and jalapeño in small amount of broth until translucent.
2. Add mushrooms and simmer to release moisture.
3. Add broth and all remaining ingredients. Cook until broccoli and vegetables are tender. Taste & adjust seasonings. Add broth to thickness preferred.
4. Add cooked noodles; heat thoroughly and serve.

OLD FASHIONED SPLIT PEA POTATO SOUP

Yield: 4 servings

This soup is surprisingly delicious! It tastes like a comforting old-fashioned meal at grandma's house!

Ingredients:

- 1 cup split peas, uncooked; rinsed & drained
- 4 cups filtered, pure water – or vegetable broth
- 1 Tbsp. Better than Vegetable Bouillon
- ½ medium onion, chopped
- 2 carrots, peeled & chopped
- 2 stalks celery, peel layer of outer strings & chop
- 2 bay leaves
- 2 – 3 tsp garlic, minced
- 2 potatoes, chopped; peeled if using russets; no need to peel red or yellow skin potatoes
- ¼ cup fresh chopped parsley
- 2 tsp basil, dried – or ¼ - ½ cup chopped fresh
- 1 tsp dried thyme, or 2 tsp fresh
- 1 tsp dried rosemary, or 2 tsp fresh
- 1 ½ tsp salt
- ½ tsp pepper, freshly ground

Directions:

1. In a large saucepan, combine the split peas, onion, bay leaves, garlic, and water.
2. Bring to a boil. Cover. Reduce heat and simmer for 2 hours. Stir occasionally.
3. Add carrots, celery, potatoes, and herbs. Simmer for 1 more hour or until peas are tender.
4. Once the peas are fully cooked and tender, add the salt and black pepper. Taste & adjust seasonings.

SPICY BEAN & SWEET POTATO SOUP

Yields: 6 - 8 servings

Sweet potato adds mellow, smooth contrast to the spices and beans. The peppers suggested in this recipe will render the soup very hot. If you do not want a HOT bean soup, omit the peppers.

Ingredients:

- ¼ - ½ cup veggie broth to sauté
- 2 - 2 ½ cups orange-fleshed sweet potatoes, peeled and cut in 1-inch cubes (*other potatoes can be used in this recipe*)
- ½ bell pepper, seeded & chopped
- 1 large onion, diced
- 1 – 2 stalks celery, diced
- 1 small can diced mild green chilies
- 1 jalapeno chili, seeded & chopped *(Omit if you don't like heat)*
- 3 large cloves garlic, minced; Or 1 Tbsp. prepared, minced garlic
- 2 – 3 tsp chili powder
- 1 – 2 tsp sweet or smoked paprika
- 2 – 3 tsp cumin
- ½ tsp nutmeg
- ½ tsp cinnamon
- ½ tsp crushed red pepper flakes (or to taste)
- 2 – 3 cups vegetable broth or water
- 1 – 28-ounce can organic crushed tomatoes
- 1 – 14-ounce can organic black beans; rinsed & drained
- 1 – 14-ounce can kidney beans; rinsed & drained
- 1 – 14-ounce can white navy beans; rinsed & drained
- 1 – 2 bay leaves
- 1 tsp Kosher, pink Himalayan or sea salt
- Ground black pepper to taste
- 3 Tbsp. freshly squeezed lime juice
- Optional: Lime wedges (for serving)

Directions:

1. In a large Dutch over, or soup pot on medium heat, add a few Tbsp. of water or vegetable broth and sauté onions, celery, chili's & bell pepper until translucent.
2. Add sweet potatoes, crushed tomatoes, garlic, salt, pepper, and spices, and broth or water, depending on which you are using, stir thoroughly and bring to a boil.
3. Reduce heat to medium-low, cover, and simmer for about 15 minutes until sweet potatoes begin to soften, stirring occasionally.
4. Add beans and continue to cook until sweet potatoes are thoroughly cooked and ready to eat.

When soup is ready to eat, stir in lime juice and serve portions with lime wedges if desired.

SIMPLE BLACK BEAN SOUP

Yields: 4 – 6 servings

Ingredients:

- 1 ½ cups dry black beans, soaked overnight or minimum of 2 hours; or use <u>Quick-Soak Method page 162.</u>
- Or, use 2; 15-ounce cans organic black beans
- 1 onion, finely chopped
- 3 cloves garlic, minced, or 1 Tbsp. minced
- 2 celery stalks, peeled & diced
- 2 carrots, peeled and diced
- ½ large red bell pepper, seeded and diced
- 1 Tbsp. ground cumin
- ¼ tsp chipotle powder or smoked paprika
- 1 - 2 large bay leaf
- 2 tsp dried oregano leaves or 2 Tbsp. fresh chopped
- ½ - 2 tsp salt, to taste
- ½ juiced fresh lemon
- 4 – 5 cups vegetable broth – watch as soup simmers and add more if necessary.

Top with a dollop of plain non-dairy yogurt.

Directions:

1. In a large Dutch oven or soup pot sauté diced onions in veggie broth until translucent.
2. Add celery and continue cooking for a few minutes.
3. Add carrots, garlic, red bell pepper and continue sautéing for another few minutes.
4. Add remaining ingredients and cook until beans are soft and ready to eat; about 30 minutes for canned beans – and approximately 1 ½ - 2 hours if using dry soaked beans.

EDD MAIN MEAL ENTRÉE SELECTIONS

If you prefer not to eat rice or potatoes – cauliflower is a great substitute with less starch and carbs. Here is a recipe for cauliflower fried rice:

CAULIFLOWER 'FRIED' RICE

Cauliflower has no real taste of its own – so it is a great base to add whatever seasonings or flavor profile you are going for.

Yields: Approximately 4 servings, depending on cauliflower size

Ingredients:

- Vegetable broth to sauté
- 1 head cauliflower
- 1 chopped onion
- 1 – 2 heaping tsp minced garlic
- Fresh herb & seasonings of choice; parsley, cilantro, tarragon, rosemary, thyme, ginger, low-sodium organic soy-sauce or Liquid Aminos, sesame oil
- Salt & fresh crushed pepper to taste

Directions:

Sauté Method;

1. Chop cauliflower into pieces, remove hard core center.
2. In food processor, pulse cauliflower with a couple quick pulses until it resembles rice. Be careful NOT to over process here. Set aside.
3. Sauté onion in small amount of vegetable broth until translucent.
4. Add minced garlic and mix until fragrance is released.
5. Depending on your chosen flavor profile, add herb – or herbs of choice. If going for oriental, add ginger, minced green onion and scant splash of toasted sesame seed oil. For savory dishes add Italian, Mexican or Indian herbs & spices per spice chart. Mix until thoroughly incorporated.
6. Top with desired vegetable, lentil or bean entrée choice.

Alternative Steam Method:

Remove core and cut cauliflower into bite-size pieces and place in steamer. Steam until tender; approximately 5 – 10 minutes. Be careful not to overcook here. You want cauliflower to maintain a crispy, yet tender texture. Think 'al dente' almost cooked, but not quite. Add herb seasoning profile of choice and top with your favorite lentil, or bean entrée mixture.

TASTY MASHED POTATOES

Yield: 6 generous servings

Ingredients:

- Depending on size of potatoes, and servings you desire to make, calculate 1 large or 2-3 small potatoes per serving. Russet, red, yellow or even sweet potatoes work for this recipe. Peeling is not necessary, but we prefer peeled mashed potatoes
- 2 Tbsp. **Better than Bouillon Organic Vegetable Base**, or equivalent
- ¼ – ½ cup non-dairy milk; unsweetened rice, or almond. Or, vegetable broth if preferred.
- ½ tsp garlic powder
- ½ tsp onion powder
- Salt & fresh ground pepper to taste

- *Optional:* Fresh herbs give these mashed potatoes extra taste. Depending on which flavor profile you are going for add a couple tablespoons of the herb of choice; parsley, tarragon, oregano, cilantro, basil, etc.

Directions:

1. Peel and boil potatoes in salted water until fork tender; approximately 10 – 15 minutes. Drain.
2. Mash potatoes with all remaining herbs and spices, adding more liquid as needed for the consistency you prefer. Serve hot & enjoy!

QUINOA PILAF

Yields: 8 servings

Quinoa adds variety to meals and contains more protein content than other grains.

Ingredients:

- 1 bell pepper, seeded & chopped
- ½ cup peeled & diced celery (*carefully peel outer layer of strings*)
- ½ cup peeled & diced carrot
- 1 Tbsp. minced garlic
- 2 tsp ground cumin
- 1 tsp dried oregano
- 2 cups quinoa, rinsed and drained
- 3 cups boiling water or vegetable broth (*add 1 tsp salt if using water or unsalted broth*)
- ¼ cup minced fresh cilantro or parsley (*optional*)

Directions:

1. In large Dutch oven, or sauce pan, broth sauté onion, celery, carrot, and garlic until they become translucent and soft.
2. Add cumin, oregano and 2 cups rinsed, drained, uncooked quinoa and cook for about 3 more minutes, stirring constantly to allow spices and quinoa to toast.
3. Add boiling salted water or vegetable broth.
4. Cover and simmer low about 20 minutes, or until all the liquid has completely absorbed and the quinoa has softened.
5. Do not stir during cooking and make sure the lid is tight to prevent moisture from escaping.
6. Remove from heat and allow quinoa to sit for 5 minutes. Add cilantro or parsley, if using. Fluff with a fork and serve.

Allow leftovers to cool and refrigerate for up to 3 days.

➢ Tip: For a variation, omit cumin and oregano and add 1 tsp dried thyme, rosemary, and/or sage for an Italian flair. Or, make it Asian, Mexican or Indian using the **Culinary Spices From Around the Word** seasoning chart.

HERB & VEGGIE BROWN RICE WITH MUSHROOMS & CAPERS

Ingredients:

- 2 cups *cooked* brown rice – or cauliflower rice
- ¼ cup vegetable broth to sauté vegetables
- ¾ cup chopped onions - about ½ large onion chopped fine
- 2 tsp minced garlic
- ½ red, orange or yellow bell pepper, seeded and diced
- 1 small zucchini chopped
- 1 cup chopped fresh mushrooms
- 1 cup chopped fresh organic spinach
- 2 Tbsp. crushed dried tarragon - or ¼ cup chopped fresh tarragon
- 2 - 3 Tbsp. capers; according to taste
- Salt & pepper to taste

Option: If you do not like capers, you can substitute with ½ cup petite green peas; frozen is fine. Add toward end of cooking time to heat up the peas; about 2 – 3 minutes.

Directions:

1. Sauté onion, bell pepper and garlic in vegetable broth until soft & translucent; approximately 3 - 4 minutes.
2. Add zucchini and cook additional 1 – 2 minutes.
3. Add mushrooms and cook until mushrooms release all of their fluid - about 3 minutes.
4. Add spinach & tarragon and cook until well mixed and heated through.
5. Add cooked brown rice or cooked cauliflower rice and mix to heat thoroughly.
6. Add capers, salt & pepper to taste and enjoy!

Tip: If rice mixture seems dry - add vegetable broth to bring it to a nice serving consistency. Add more vegetables to make this a nutritious, delicious meal.

MEXICAN LENTIL CHILI

Yields: 4 - 6 servings

Ingredients:

- 1 ½ cups organic lentils
- 2 15 oz. cans organic fire roasted or regular diced tomatoes
- 1 large carrot peeled and diced
- 6 cups vegetable broth - or water - or a combination of both
- 1 Tbsp. cumin
- 1 Tbsp. red chili powder
- ½ tsp cayenne powder - or hot pepper sauce of your choice
- 1 Tbsp. minced garlic
- 1 small onion diced
- 1 small can diced green chilies - or 1 diced, seeded green chili
- ¼ cup diced fresh cilantro
- 1 tsp pink salt
- black pepper to taste

Directions:

1. Rinse and drain lentils.
2. Add all ingredients to large pot and bring to a boil. Turn to low and simmer, covered for approximately 1 hour.
3. Directions on the lentil bag says 40 - 50 minutes to cook, but my experience is lentils take much longer to cook - AND - lentils are VERY thirsty! So be watchful and add more liquid as necessary.
4. Cook lentils until soft, yummy and ready to eat!

➤ **Tip:** Eat alone or pour chili over your favorite rice or quinoa dish, or couple it with the Mexican Butternut Squash.

POTATO CAULIFLOWER CURRY

Yields: 6 servings

Turmeric and other Indian spices are getting more and more attention for their anticancer properties. For a hotter curry, increase the amount of cayenne. This tasty curry can be poured over brown rice, mashed potatoes or Quinoa Pilaf.

Ingredients:

- ¼ - ½ cup veggie broth
- 1 onion, chopped or thinly sliced
- 1 15-ounce can chopped tomatoes, or 1 1/2 cups freshly chopped tomatoes
- ¼ tsp cayenne – or ½ tsp garlic chili paste
- ¼ tsp cinnamon
- ¼ tsp ground ginger
- ½ tsp ground coriander
- ½ tsp turmeric
- 1 tsp curry powder
- 1 tsp cumin seeds; *toasted if desired.* Or, 1 – 2 tsp powder cumin
- 1 head cauliflower, cut into bite-size florets; hard center core removed
- 2 medium potatoes, chopped and peeled
- ½ - 1 tsp salt to taste

Directions:

1. Broth sauté onion over medium-high heat for about 3 minutes, until translucent.
2. Reduce heat to medium, add potatoes and cauliflower. Continue cooking, stirring often, for about 5 minutes. Add water or broth, ¼ cup at a time, as needed to prevent sticking.
3. Toast cumin seeds, turmeric, coriander, ginger, cinnamon, and cayenne in a dry skillet over medium heat for about 2 minutes, stirring constantly. Add spices to vegetables along with tomatoes, and salt. Stir to mix, then cover and simmer for about 20 minutes until flavors are blended. Serve & enjoy!

THAI VEGGIE SAUTÉ

Yields: 8 servings *(this recipe can be easily halved)*

Ingredients:

- 2 Tbsp. minced garlic
- 2 Tbsp. minced ginger
- 2 Tbsp. fresh mint
- 2 Tbsp. fresh basil
- 2 Tbsp. fresh cilantro
- 2 carrots peeled and grated
- 2 – 3 cups vegetable broth
- 1 tsp toasted sesame seed oil
- 1 bell pepper, seeded and chopped
- 1 large eggplant, peeled, cut into 1 inch cubes
- 2 cups green beans, cut in 2 inch pieces
- 3 cups mushrooms; try a blend of oriental shitake & oyster
- 2 Tbsp. Better Than Vegetable Bouillon
- 1 tsp curry powder
- ½ cup unsweetened coconut milk
- ½ cup dry toasted hulled sunflower seeds

Directions:

1. Use a large Wok – or a very large Dutch oven skillet. Add all ingredients except the coconut milk & toasted sunflower seeds.
2. Bring to a boil, cover and simmer, stirring occasionally, until all the vegetables are tender.
3. Taste, adjust seasonings, add coconut milk & toasted sunflower seeds. Serve & enjoy!

LOUSIANA STYLE RED BEANS & RICE

This is one of our go to all-time favorites – especially for the EDD. Make up a big batch of this luscious food and eat it for a couple days for mid-day meals or supper. Bon Appetite!

Yields: 4 - 6 servings

Ingredients:

- 2 cups dried red kidney beans; soaked overnight, or using the Quick-Soak Method page 162. Or, four 15-ounce cans, or two large 28 ounce cans
- 1 large bell pepper; seeded and chopped
- 1 large onion; chopped small
- 3 large carrots; peeled & diced
- 3 large celery stalks; peeled & diced
- 4 – 5 cups low-sodium, organic vegetable broth
- 3 bay leaves
- 2 heaping Tbsp. minced garlic
- 2 Tbsp. Better than Bouillon Organic Vegetable Base
- 2 tsp cumin
- 1 tsp Kosher, or sea salt, or pink Himalayan salt
- Cracked black pepper to taste
- 2 cups cooked white, brown or cauliflower rice - prepared according to package *(Cauliflower Rice; page 213)*.
- *Optional:* Tabasco, Siracha, or Louisiana Red Pepper Sauce

  - ➤ **Tip:** These beans are also wonderful poured over the top of the grain of your choice; quinoa, wild rice, millet, or a nice grain combo.

Directions:

1. Sauté onions, celery and bell pepper in a couple tablespoons of vegetable broth. As they cook, add 1 teaspoon of salt, and sweat the vegetables until transparent; adding small amounts of broth if necessary to not burn the vegetables. Be careful not to allow them to brown.
2. Add carrots, bay leaves and garlic, stirring to mix well.
3. Add beans, cumin, bullion, salt, pepper and broth.

4. If using canned beans, cover and cook for approximately 30 - 40 minutes - until carrots are very soft.
5. If using soaked, dried beans, cook for approximately 2 - 3 hours, until beans are tender and cooked thoroughly.
6. Pour mixture over hot cooked rice, or cooked grain of your choice.

A few splashes of Tabasco, or your favorite Louisiana hot sauce goes very well here!

LENTIL ARTICHOKE STEW

Yields: 4 - 6 Servings

This aromatic Middle Eastern dish is great served alone or over brown rice or quinoa pilaf. Using fire-roasted tomatoes is not essential, but they will give the stew a delicious smoky flavor.

Ingredients:
- ¼ cup vegetable broth
- ¼ tsp salt
- ¼ tsp crushed red pepper (optional)
- 3 - 4 Tbsp. freshly squeezed lemon juice
- 1 cup quartered canned or thawed frozen artichoke hearts or bottoms. *(We prefer canned artichoke bottoms rather than hearts; less shredded fiber in stew)*
- 2 24-ounce cans chopped, organic fire-roasted tomatoes, undrained, or 6 cups chopped fresh tomatoes plus 1 cup vegetable broth
- 1 – 2 bay leaves
- 1 cup dry red lentils
- 2 cups water or vegetable broth
- 1 tsp ground coriander
- 2 tsp ground cumin
  2 large garlic cloves, minced or pressed
- 1 onion, chopped
- ¼ tsp ground black pepper

Directions:
1. Broth sauté onion over medium heat for about 5 minutes, until translucent.
2. Add the garlic, cumin, and coriander and cook for 2 minutes, stirring frequently.
3. Add the water or vegetable broth, lentils, and bay leaf and bring to a boil.
4. Reduce the heat and add the tomatoes and their liquid, the artichoke hearts, lemon juice, and optional red pepper flakes. Simmer for about 20 - 40 minutes, or until the lentils are tender. Remove and discard the bay leaf. Season with salt and pepper to taste.

MUSHROOM LENTIL BOURUIGNON

Yields: 4 – 6 servings

This delicious lentil dish is fantastic over mashed potatoes. It provides a satisfying mouthful of textures between the chewy mushrooms and lentils, over smooth mashed potatoes. Yum!

Ingredients:

- 1 cup dry lentils
- 4 cups vegetable broth (*After EDD use 1 cup red wine and 3 cups broth*)
- 2 – 3 cups assorted mushrooms; Portobello, shitake, oyster, cremini
- ½ large onion, chopped
- 1 Tbsp. Better Than Vegetable Bouillon
- 1 – 2 Tbsp. minced garlic; to taste
- 1 Tbsp. dried thyme; or ¼ cup diced fresh
- 1 Tbsp. dried tarragon; or ¼ cup diced fresh
- ¼ cup chopped fresh parsley
- 1 tsp pink salt, Kosher or sea salt
- 3 bay leaves
- 1 Tbsp. tomato paste
- Crushed black pepper to taste
- Option: 1 – 2 Tbsp. gluten-free flour

Directions:

1. Sauté onion and garlic in vegetable broth until translucent.
2. Add all remaining ingredients, bring to a boil, turn down heat, cover and cook until lentils are tender about 45 minutes or longer depending on what type of lentils you use.
3. Lentils can be thirsty, so check on liquid level and adjust as needed.
4. If stew seems watery, add a couple tablespoons of gluten-free flour such as tapioca flour.
5. When cooked, remove bay leaves and serve over mashed potatoes.

MEXICAN BUTTERNUT SQUASH

Yields: Approximately 4 servings

Ingredients:

- 1 organic butternut squash; seeded, cooked & mashed
- ¼ cup vegetable broth for sautéing
- 1 can organic black beans
- 1 medium purple onion, diced
- 1 mild green chili, seeded and diced. Or, 1 small can diced green chilies
- 2 cups fresh organic spinach chopped
- ½ cup diced bell pepper
- ½ cup organic cilantro
- 1 fresh lime juiced
- 1 tsp paprika - sweet or smoked - your preference
- 2 tsp chili powder
- 2 tsp whole cumin seeds - pan roasted. Or, 2 – 3 tsp cumin powder
- 1 heaping Tbsp. minced garlic
- ½ tsp pink salt
- ½ tsp white pepper - or fresh black pepper to taste

Option: **After** EDD add 1 cup organic frozen - or canned - sweet corn

Directions:

Preheat oven to 400 degrees.

1. Rinse and slice butternut squash in half length-wise. Use a very sharp knife - be careful - these suckers are very hard to cut, remove seeds.
2. Place cut side down on a cookie sheet lined with parchment paper. Bake for about 60 minutes. Cook until soft and thoroughly cooked through.
3. Once butternut squash is soft & cooked, scoop out soft flesh and discard outer skin layer and set aside.
4. While squash is baking, roast cumin seeds in a small dry, non-stick fry pan until brown and fragrant. Be watchful and continue lifting, flipping and stirring - be careful not to scorch. These seeds smell fantastic! Toast and set aside.

5. In medium saucepan sauté onions & bell peppers in veggie broth until soft and translucent. If using fresh mild green chili add now with onion and bell pepper and cook until translucent.
6. Add garlic and cook until fragrant.
7. Add spinach & and stir until thoroughly incorporated.
8. Add cilantro & mix thoroughly.
9. Add all remaining ingredients; canned green chilies if using, black beans, roasted cumin seeds, paprika, chili powder, salt, lime and pepper to taste and heat thoroughly.
10. Add squash and mix to heat thoroughly.
11. Taste again and season according to your personal preference.

Top with fresh squeezed lime for an additional burst of flavor.

➢ Tip: This delicious **Mexican Butternut Squash** can be served with a nice green leafy salad, or broth-sautéed vegetable side dish or paired with **Mexican Lentil Chili** - we have paired these two recipes many times.

➢ This delicious mixture makes an AWESOME filling for enchiladas! Check out my recipe for **Mexican Butternut Squash Enchiladas** in the *After EDD Recipe Section*.

<u>EASY DELICIOUS SIMPLE QUINOA CHILI</u>

Yields: 6 - 8 servings

Ingredients:

- 1 cup organic quinoa cooked according to package directions; yields 2 cups cooked grain
- ¼ - ½ cup vegetable broth to sauté
- 1 can organic black beans
- 1 can organic kidney beans
- 1 small onion, diced
- 2 14.5 ounce cans organic fire roasted or regular diced tomatoes
- 1 small can diced green chilies; or 1 fresh chili seeded and chopped
- 5 green onions, diced
- ½ cup chopped fresh cilantro
- 1 cup organic; low sodium vegetable broth
- 1 Tbsp. minced garlic
- 1 tsp crushed oregano
- 2 Tbsp. red chili powder
- 2 Tbsp. cumin powder
- 2 tsp Ancho chili powder - or hot chili sauce or Cayenne powder according to your taste
- 2 tsp pink salt
- Crushed black pepper

Directions:

1. Cook quinoa according to package directions.
2. While quinoa is cooking sauté onion & minced garlic in broth until very soft and cooked thoroughly. You don't want crunchy onions in your chili. If they seem to become dry, add a small amount of vegetable broth to soften and continue cooking.
3. Add green onions and cook to blend & soften another 1-2 minutes.
4. Add green chilies & fresh cilantro, stir to blend.

5. Add the 1 cup vegetable broth, 2 cans of fire roasted tomatoes, black beans and kidney beans and the spices and mix thoroughly. Cook 10 - 15 minutes to allow spices and ingredients to blend well and soften the beans.
6. At this point taste your tomato, bean, spice mixture and add more seasoning if you desire. Cook until vegetables are soft and cooked thoroughly.
7. Add cooked quinoa - mix thoroughly and heat through. Add more broth if necessary to make a nice, thick chili consistency.
8. Taste & adjust seasons and serve.

Serve with a little fresh lime & extra chili sauce if desired and enjoy!!!

SAVORY LENTIL SOUP

Yields: 4 servings

This recipe can easily be doubled for more servings. Cooking time for lentils varies. If you choose to soak the lentils, cooking time will be reduced. Soaking is not necessary, but it does help with digestion, and cuts down on cooking time.

Ingredients:

- 1 cup dried lentils (soak 24 hours for shorter cooking time; *but not required*)
- 1 onion, chopped
- 3 carrots, peeled and diced
- 3 large celery stalks, diced (*peel outside strings for more enjoyable texture)*
- 4 cups low-sodium organic vegetable broth (*more if necessary for consistency*)
- 1 14.5 oz can diced tomatoes, try organic, Muir Glenn fire roasted for a special treat. Or, 1 - 2 diced fresh, organic tomatoes
- 2 tsp. Kosher, sea salt, or pink Himalayan salt
- 2 – 3 bay leaves
- 1 tsp. cumin powder
- 1 tsp. coriander powder

Directions:

1. Sauté onions and celery in 2 – 3 tablespoons of vegetable broth - add the salt & "sweat" cook until soft & translucent. Do not brown.
2. When vegetables are translucent, add all remaining ingredients, cover and cook approximately 45 minutes, checking to see when lentils become soft, and all vegetables cook thoroughly.
3. If you choose, and have an immersion blender, you can immerse the blender into the soup and "mulch" it to a nice, thick, chunky consistency.
4. Or, you can pour 1/2 the soup into a blender, or food processor, and blend or process until smooth and then pour blended soup back into the remaining lentil soup for a pleasant chunky, smooth texture.
5. Taste and adjust seasoning as desired.

INDIAN-SPICED VEGGIE MEDLEY

Yields: 4 - 6 servings

Choose your favorite vegetables here – below is a suggestion, but use what you have on hand.

Ingredients:

- ¼ cup vegetable broth to sauté
- 1 onion, diced
- 1 bell pepper chopped
- ½ cup chopped parsley, or cilantro
- 1 green chili or jalapeno, seeded and diced *(4 oz. small can green chilies)*
- 2 cups vegetable broth
- 1 15 oz. can diced tomatoes; include liquid
- 1 cup fresh green beans, if in season
- 1 small zucchini chopped
- 2 – 3 tsp minced garlic
- 1 tsp mustard seed
- 1 tsp cumin seed
- 1 tsp sweet or smoked paprika
- 1 tsp turmeric powder
- 1 tsp curry powder
- 1 tsp cardamom
- 1 tsp ground coriander
- 1 tsp pink, Kosher, or sea salt

Directions:

1. Toast dry mustard & cumin seeds in small non-stick pan, careful not to burn. Once toasted, remove from heat and set aside.
2. Sauté onion and bell pepper in vegetable broth until translucent.
3. Add all remaining ingredients and cook until vegetables are tender.

Variations: You can pour this veggie medley over rice, mashed potatoes or favorite cooked grain. Or, just enjoy as is!

DELICIOUS GLUTEN-FREE VEGAN PIZZA

> ➤ **Tip:** While on the EDD, cashews are not actually 'legal' ... *however*... a small amount on top of this delicious GF vegan pizza is a fun 'splurge' and well worth the effort in making it. Cashew cream – in the future – is a much healthier choice than dairy cow cheese.

Yield: 2 Medium-large pizza's

If you have a pizza stone – use it. You will need parchment paper & rolling pin to create this GF pizza crust.

This pizza is a little labor intensive, but it is fun and worth it. Choose a lazy weekend afternoon and dig in. It is well worth the effort.

GF Pizza Crust Ingredients:

- 2 2/3 cups gluten-free flour such as *Pamela's Artisan Certified non-GMO Gluten-Free* flour, or Bob Red Mill's organic gluten-free flour. Or, quinoa flour.
- 2 tsp yeast
- 1 Tbsp. psyllium husk for extra fiber
- 1 tsp pink, Kosher or sea salt
- 1 cup cooked, mashed potato
- 1 ¼ cup reserved warm starchy water

Italian Pizza Sauce:

- ¼ cup vegetable broth
- ¼ onion, diced
- 2 tsp minced garlic
- 1 tsp dried oregano
- 1 tsp dried basil
- 1 tsp dried parsley
- 1 tsp dried thyme
- ½ tsp salt
- 1 15 oz. can organic tomato sauce
- 1 15 oz. can organic diced tomatoes – drained

- 1 tsp raw honey, or pure maple syrup

Sauce Directions:

1. In saucepan sauté onion and minced garlic in small amount of vegetable broth until translucent.
2. Add tomato sauce, diced tomatoes and all herbs and spices.
3. Cook covered while preparing the rest of the pizza.
4. Taste, adjust seasonings and top pizza when ready.

Vegan Cashew Cheese:

- ½ cup raw cashew nuts, soaked in boiling water for at least 15 minutes; then drain.
- 1 cup unsweetened rice or almond milk
- 1 Tbsp. fresh squeezed lemon *(or more to taste)*
- ¼ tsp garlic powder
- 1 tsp dried tarragon
- Scant dash of salt
- 1 Tbsp. Nutritional Yeast
- 2 Tbsp. Tapioca starch

Cashew Cheese Directions:

1. Place soaked, drained cashews, non-dairy milk, lemon, garlic powder, tarragon, salt & tapioca starch into a small food processor or heavy-duty blender and mix until thoroughly liquefied.
2. In a small saucepan, bring cashew mixture to a gentle boil, cooking a few minutes to heat, then add Nutritional Yeast and cook and stir to blend thoroughly.
3. Cook until mixture thickens. Once nice and thick, cover and turn off heat. If mixture becomes too thick, thin with small amount of vegetable broth until it is of 'scoop able' consistency. Scoop in small spoonful's onto pizza just before final cooking with sauce and toppings.

Pizza Crust Directions:

1. Boil 2 – 3 small potatoes until fork tender; reserve starchy liquid. You can keep peel on until boiled, then it is easy to skin. Or peel before cooking.
2. Mash potato thoroughly and measure out one cup.
3. In a small bowl, activate the 2 tsp yeast in a couple tablespoons of the warm starchy water. It will begin to bubble when activated.
4. Mix flour with salt and psyllium husk thoroughly.
5. Using a spatula add activated yeast and mashed potato to flour mixture.
6. Mix the dough as best you can to incorporate, flipping with the spatula and working the flour into the potatoes.
7. Now begin to incorporate starchy water – start with one cup and slowly work up until you have a very thick batter – you do not want it too wet – you will need to mix with your hands; slightly dampen your palms if necessary.
8. When you can form the dough into a large round mound – separate in two, cover with plastic and let rest at least 30 minutes.

Dough will be thick and sticky. Don't worry, gluten-free pizza dough is goopy in texture. This dough will stick to the parchment paper completely, but once the crust is cooked the paper comes right off without sticking.

If you desire – refrigerate half of this pizza dough in air tight container for up to 3 days and then prepare as directed.

Rolling out Pizza Dough:

1. After dough rests 30 minutes to an hour – cut two large equal-sized pieces of parchment paper.
2. Place dough in center of first piece of parchment paper and top with second piece of equal size.
3. Carefully roll out dough between the two sheets. Now, the sheets will want to wrinkle, so don't roll too hard. Be careful to avoid deep wrinkles in the parchment paper as it puts uneven slits in the crust. When wrinkles begin to form, very gently pull on sides of parchment to release any wrinkles. Turnover and do the same with the other side; flipping back and forth rolling carefully until a large, thin, even dough is formed. This may sound

complicated, but as you begin to roll, you will see what I mean. You'll get the hang of it.

Cooking Directions:

Preheat oven to 500 degrees. If you have a pizza stone use it.

1. Place parchment wrapped pizza dough directly onto the heated pizza stone, or place it on a pizza pan, or large cookie sheet.
2. Cook crust for 10 minutes.
3. Pull out of oven and check to see if parchment paper will come off easily. If it DOES NOT pop off instantly, set back into oven and cook additional 1 – 2 minutes until paper comes off easily.
4. Remove paper and return crust to oven and cook additional 5 minutes directly on stone, or pizza pan.
5. When crust appears nicely brown and seemingly cooked through, remove crust and spread with favorite toppings:
   a. Layer with Italian Sauce, or Marinara, or other favorite sauce.
   b. Drop Cashew Cheese over pizza in small spoonful's.
   c. Top with vegetables; onions, mushroom, bell peppers, black olives, fresh basil, fresh spinach, etc.
6. Return to oven placing directly on stone, or pizza pan and cook additional 5 – 10 minutes until toppings are cooked through.

Slice and enjoy!

KUNG PAO CAULIFLOWER STIR-FRY

Yields: Approximately 4 – 5 servings

This Kung Pao sauce is delicious and works with whatever ingredients you want to use for a fun, authentic Chinese flair!

Cauliflower Ingredients:

- ¼ cup low-sodium organic vegetable broth for sautéing
- 1 head cauliflower*, cored and chopped into florets
- 1 – 2 large carrot peeled and grated
- 2 tablespoons dry sherry
- 2 tablespoons organic low-sodium soy sauce or Liquid Aminos
- 2 tsp fresh garlic
- 2 tsp fresh ginger
- 5 diced green onions
- 1 Tbsp. tapioca starch (*tapioca flour and starch are the same*)
- ½ tsp salt
- ¼ tsp white pepper
- ½ tsp cayenne pepper flakes (*more if you like heat*)
- *Optional:* ¾ cup dry roasted husked sunflower seeds (*After EDD; peanuts*)

Kung Pao Sauce Ingredients:

- 4 Tbsp. organic low-sodium soy sauce or Liquid Aminos
- 2 Tbsp. white wine vinegar
- 2 Tbsp. dry sherry
- 1 tsp toasted sesame seed oil
- 1 ½ cups low sodium organic vegetable broth
- 2 Tbsp. coconut sugar
- 2 Tbsp. tapioca starch (*or, after EDD cornstarch*)
- ½ tsp white pepper
- ½ tsp garlic chili sauce (*less or more depending on your heat preference*)
- ½ tsp salt

Directions:

1. Combine all cauliflower stir-fry ingredients in a bowel and let marinate while you make the sauce and toast the sunflower seeds – if using.
2. Dry roast sunflower seeds in non-stick pan until golden brown, be careful not to burn. Set aside.
3. For sauce mix all ingredients in a saucepan and cook over medium heat until thick and bubbly.
4. Heat wok or large non-stick frying pan. Pour enough broth to stir-fry cauliflower vegetable mixture. Cook cauliflower & vegetables until tender, stirring often.
5. Once vegetables are tender and ready to eat, pour hot Kung Poa sauce over vegetables, add roasted sunflower seeds.
6. Pour over your favorite rice or cooked grains** and enjoy!

➢ **Tip:** *Cauliflower Substitution:* After the EDD, follow the exact recipe and substitute the cauliflower for *organic* tofu, chicken, shrimp or beef for an authentic tasting Kung Poa dish.

➢ **Tip:** **After the EDD: This Kung Pao recipe works wonderfully with oriental Pad Thai noodles. Cook one 8 oz. package of organic noodles according to package directions, rinse and drain. Once the Kung Pao vegetables are cooked and you have added the sauce, add the cooked noodles directly to the pan of Kung Pao and mix thoroughly to heat the noodles. Serve and enjoy!

- AFTER EDD -

FOOD RE-INTRODUCTION

Slowly Re-Introduce Eliminated Foods

After the 21-day Elimination Detox Diet, add one single eliminated food at a time. Wait four days to add an additional eliminated food. If you add two or more eliminated foods back into your diet at the same time – and symptoms re-occur, you will not know which of the foods are causing you distress.

Sometimes it takes up to four days for symptoms to re-occur. If symptoms reappear, eliminate this food once again. Once you are symptom free, introduce another eliminated food. If symptoms do not appear in four days, this food is acceptable to begin eating again. If symptoms re-appear, eliminate this food also. Continue this process, always being aware of your body speak symptoms. Your body will tell you which foods are OK and which are not.

During this time continue to work on healing your gut with pro-biotics, fermented foods and eating clean, organic foods. Wait another month or two and try one of the eliminated foods again and see if the symptoms re-occur. Keep up this routine until you either heal your gut enough to add these foods back into your diet, or know that this food must remain eliminated for now.

Due to the adaptive immune system's memory, it may take your body six months to a year or more to allow foods to be eaten that previously caused an immune reaction response. It is possible to heal your gut enough to reintroduce some or all of these foods back into your diet. You may also discover that some foods must be permanently eliminated from your diet.

Mental Attitude & Intentionality

Be patient. You have come this far, go slow and take it easy. If you rush this process you are in danger of ending up back where you began. Some of my clients and students have 'crawled' through the food elimination process focusing on what they cannot eat, feeling like a victim and as soon as the 21-days end – they race off to fast-food restaurants and instantly add *everything* back into their diet, undoing whatever good they did. All symptoms returned with a vengeance because the body did not have enough time to heal itself.

Others have embraced the 21-day EDD and are now living a full plant-based diet free of processed and animal foods. They are enjoying vibrancy, energy and experiencing no digestive distress whatsoever. They are listening to their bodies, employing the skills they learned through this program and are thriving, healthy, strong and loving their lives every day. You can too!

You and your body deserve to heal and enjoy life. Take it easy, live careful, aware and intentional. Continue to hone your Body Speak skills. Don't stop – ever. This is just the beginning. Living intentional and in-tune with your body will empower you to achieve all of your health goals. It is within your power to achieve and maintain health and enjoy life to its fullest.

Where To Go Now?

Now that you've read through all the Why's and How's of this book, it's time to determine what road is best for you moving forward. A plant-based diet? An animal food diet? Or a combination of mostly plants, with a little organic grass-fed animal food. The choice is yours.

Hopefully, you have successfully traversed through the 'elimination' diet and understand now if there are foods that are causing you digestive issues. I hope you tried all of these recipes and understand how delicious, nutritious and satisfying whole foods are. Even vegan meals! Who knew?

Foods to Add – Foods to Avoid

The foods you have eliminated during the EDD are foods that can remain permanently eliminated if you choose. There is no *need* to eat soy, eggs, sugar, beef, chicken, fish or oil to maintain optimal health.

Soy: If you choose to eat soy, eat fermented only.

Eggs: If you choose to eat eggs, eat only cage-free organic eggs in moderation. There is controversy over the health benefits of eggs. Egg yolks contain cholesterol and may contribute to plaque build-up in the body. If you like eggs and have no adverse Body Speak reactions after re-introducing them back into your diet – then enjoy!

Oil is Saturated Fat:

"The fat you eat is the fat you wear,"
Dr. John McDougall, physician, author and nutrition expert.

Dr. McDougall's plant-based food protocol has healed thousands of people for over forty years. I respect this healing doctor and I hear his words in my head every time I plop a tablespoon of coconut oil in a pan or use it in baked goods. I do not want to wear fat of any kind. I have cut way down on using coconut oil – even though many health practitioners do not have an issue with using it. I believe caution and moderation is key here.

Using Oil: Use sparingly, if at all. Oil is an isolated food with no nutritional value. Use only organic oil. On EDD, you have learned how to sauté exclusively in water or vegetable broth, it is a healthy choice to continue to do so.

Coconut Oil: Coconut oil comes in two forms; refined, which means it has no coconut taste, and virgin which means the flavor is maintained. Refined coconut oil is good for sautéing foods as it does not add coconut flavor. Baking with virgin coconut oil does add the coconut flavor, but in some cases this enhances the flavor of baked goods.

Healthy Fats: The healthy fats to add into your diet are avocadoes, nuts and seeds. Nut butters in baked goods work great to moisten foods, add protein and flavor.

The following chapter contains a selection of our favorite gluten-free and vegan 'go-to' recipes. Some of these recipes include oil, corn, nuts and eggs, so be sure you have successfully traversed the EDD re-introduction protocol before adding them back into your diet.

In the list of **Resources, Chapter 20**, you will find a list of reliable sources for healing physicians, detox specialists, overcoming cancer experts, and trustworthy, reliable laboratories offering high-grade 'nutraceutical' supplements to enhance and upgrade your journey of recovery and thriving health.

Chapter 19

AFTER EDD

DELICIOUS HEALTHY RECIPES

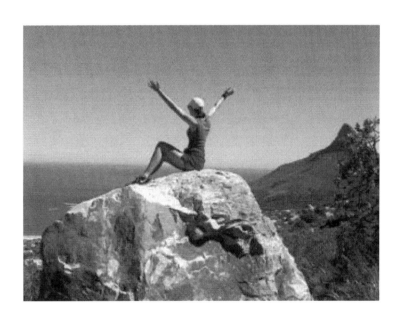

A Few Favorite Go-to Recipes

GLUTEN FREE CINNAMON NUT BREAD

Yields: One loaf of bread - about 12 slices.

I like to slice this bread and wrap it in plastic and freeze it. It makes wonderful toast topped with homemade applesauce.

Ingredients:

Dry:

- 1 cup sunflower seeds *(mixed in food processor until crumpled & almost powdery)*
- ½ cup flax seeds
- 1 cup almonds *(mixed in food processor to medium - small chunks)*
- 1 ½ cups organic rolled oats
- ½ cup shredded unsweetened coconut
- 2 Tbsp. chia seeds
- 4 Tbsp. psyllium seed husks *(3 Tbsp. if using psyllium husk powder)*
- 1 tsp fine grain sea salt *(add 1/2 tsp if using coarse salt such as pink Himalayan or Kosher)*
- 2 tsp cinnamon
- 1 tsp nutmeg
- ½ tsp allspice

Wet:

- 2 Tbsp. maple syrup - or honey
- 2 Tbsp. melted coconut oil
- 1 Tbsp. pure vanilla
- 1 ½ cups water

Directions:

1. Spray the bottom & sides of a loaf pan with coconut oil.
2. Cut two strips of parchment paper slightly overlapping the width of your loaf pan. Place the two strips crisscross onto the pan – overlapping the pan to

make handles to easily remove later on. Press the parchment paper down onto the sprayed pan, and it will stick to it fairly well. The sheets of parchment paper act as "handles" to remove this bread 1/2 way through the cooking process, so make sure they overlap the edges of the pan on two sides. When bread mixture is ready you will press it into this prepared pan.

3. Use a small food processor to process sunflower seeds until they are uniformly crumbled. Remove sunflower seeds and add the cup of almonds to the same processor and process almonds until they are medium chunks.

4. Add all dry ingredients including spices in mixing bowl and stir to mix thoroughly.

5. **Mix together all wet ingredients** in a large two cup measuring cup until thoroughly blended and pour wet mixture over the top of the dry ingredients and combine thoroughly.

6. Press the bread mixture into the bottom of your prepared loaf pan.

7. **Cover lightly with saran and let rest for a minimum of two hours.** This bread is full of fiber and this two-hour rest time allows the water to absorb into the fiber.

8. After bread rests for two hours – or overnight – Bake in 350 F. degree oven for 20 - 30 minutes. Remove from the oven and carefully using your parchment paper "handles" remove bread from the loaf pan.

9. Place partially cooked bread loaf onto a baking rack and place directly onto the middle rack in the oven and continue cooking for an additional 30 to 40 minutes.

Bread is done when it has a nice crunchy exterior and sounds slightly "hollow" when tapped.

Allow bread to cool thoroughly, slice and serve!

Suggestion: *Serve it with Raw Apple Compote, page 186.*

GLUTEN FREE OAT PANCAKES

Yields: about 12 pancakes; *batter saves well refrigerated in air-tight container for up to 2 days*

Ingredients:

- ¾ cup organic oat flour. *(It is hard to find organic so I grind ¾ cup organic steel-cut oats in my coffee grinder. It works great.*
- ¾ cup organic non-gluten flour; i.e. teff, quinoa, millet or Pamela's artisan blend *(if you can't find quinoa flour, grind regular quinoa in a coffee grinder)*
- 1 tsp baking soda
- 1 tsp baking powder
- 1 tsp cinnamon
- ½ tsp pure vanilla extract
- ½ tsp sea salt
- ¼ cup pure maple syrup, or raw honey
- 1 ½ cups non-dairy milk; coconut or almond
- 2 Tbsp. coconut oil
- Vegan option: 2 Tbsp. flaxseed meal (ground flaxseed) plus 2 Tbsp. water
- Non vegan option: two eggs

Directions:

1. For vegan flax eggs; combine ground flaxseed & water in a cup and let sit for about 5 minutes to thicken.
2. Combine all dry ingredients.
3. Combine all wet ingredients; including eggs or flaxseed mixture, whisk to blend.
4. Combine wet & dry ingredients. Let batter sit for about 5 minutes to thicken.
5. Heat griddle and cook pancakes in a small amount of coconut oil. Oat flour takes a little longer to cook than regular gluten wheat flour. Oat pancakes brown quickly, so it is easy to over-brown the outside and undercook the center. It's best to cook on medium heat being careful to cook all the way through before serving. Use a loose fitting lid to help the cooking process.

VEGAN MAC N' CHEESE

Yields: 4 servings

This creamy satisfying gluten-free, dairy free pasta dish makes a good base for a variety of pasta dishes. Using this plain base recipe, I have created **Italian Mac n' Cheese** *(page 243). And chilled* **Potluck Pasta Salad** *(page 245). Experiment with your favorite flavors and enjoy!*

Basic – Plain - Vegan Mac N' Cheese Ingredients:

- 1 cup raw cashews; pour boiling water over cashews and let soak a minimum of 15 minutes
- 1 cup vegetable broth
- 1 ½ cups water
- ¼ cup nutritional yeast
- 2 tsp sea salt
- 2 Tbsp. fresh lemon or lime juice
- 1 Tbsp. apple cider vinegar
- 12 ounces gluten-free pasta

Basic Vegan Mac N' Cheese Directions:

1. Cook pasta according to package directions; drain and set aside.
2. Drain cashews and discard soaking water. In a high-speed blender combine cashews, 2 cups vegetable broth, nutritional yeast, salt, vinegar and lemon juice. Blend until completely smooth. Using a spatula scrape cashew cream into a sauce pan.
3. Pour 1 cup water into the blender and pulse a few times to gather up all remaining bits of cashew cream and add to sauce pan. Cover and turn heat on low. Once cashew cream is warm and slightly thickened add it to the recipe of your choice.

Plain Vegan Mac N' Cheese: Once cashew cream is warm and thickened, add it directly to the cooked drained pasta, heat through and serve. <u>Option:</u> Add a dash of nutmeg for an old-world taste.

ITALIAN MAC N' CHEESE

*Follow directions for Basic – Plain **Vegan Mac N' Cheese** (page 243) – **AND** –*
Add the following herbs & spices to the Cashew Cream Mixture:

- 1 Tbsp. dried parsley
- 1 Tbsp. dry oregano
- 1 Tbsp. onion powder
- 1 Tbsp. dry basil
- 1 tsp granulated onion powder
- 1 tsp granulated garlic powder
- 1 tsp nutmeg; *adds rich, deep flavor*

Italian Vegetable Medley Ingredients:

- 1 small onion, diced
- 1 small zucchini, or one cup broccoli florets, chopped
- 1 cup mushrooms, sliced
- ½ bell pepper, seeded & chopped
- 1 Tbsp. Better Than Vegetable Bouillon
- 1 Tbsp. minced garlic
- 1 cup vegetable broth
- ¼ cup fresh chopped parsley
- 1 Tbsp. dry basil, or ¼ cup fresh
- 2 tsp dry oregano, or 2 Tbsp. fresh
- 1 tsp rosemary
- 1 tsp salt
- Crushed black pepper to taste - *optional*

Italian Mac N' Cheese Directions:

1. *Pasta:* Make basic Vegan Mac N' Cheese – **adding above herbs & spices.**
2. *Italian Vegetables:* Sauté onion, bell pepper and garlic until translucent.
3. Add remaining vegetable ingredients and cook until vegetables are tender and ready to eat.
4. Add the Italian vegetable medley to the Italian Mac N' Cheese heat through and serve.

POTLUCK PASTA SALAD

Prepare one batch of Basic Vegan Mac N' Cheese using gluten-free elbow macaroni or small shell pasta. Chop up your favorite pasta salad vegetables and add 1 – 2 Tbsp. of your favorite oil-free salad dressing; add it all together, chill and enjoy. Below are the vegetables we like to use in pasta salad.

Ingredients:

- ½ cup sliced black olives
- ½ cup sliced pimento stuffed green olives
- 2 green onions diced
- ½ chopped bell pepper
- 1 cup chopped broccoli florets
- 2 Tbsp. sweet pickle relish
- 1 tsp onion powder
- 1 Tbsp. tarragon
- 1 Tbsp. rice wine vinegar
- 1 Tbsp. raw honey
- 1 tsp salt
- Crushed black pepper to taste; *optional*

OUTSTANDING HOME-MADE ENCHILADA SAUCE

Yields: 2 ½ cups – Easily doubles for larger batches

Ingredients:

- 2 Tbsp. extra virgin organic olive oil
- 2 Tbsp. gluten-free all-purpose flour
- 2 Tbsp. red chili powder
- 1 Tbsp. granulated onion powder *(not onion salt)*
- 2 tsp cumin powder
- 1 tsp garlic powder
- 1 tsp smoked or sweet paprika
- ¼ tsp cayenne, or other hot chili powder
- ½ tsp raw honey
- 1 ½ cups low sodium organic vegetable broth
- 1 small can organic tomato paste

Directions:

1. Add olive oil to sauce pan and turn on heat. Whisk the gluten-free flour into the oil and stir until flour is smooth and lump-free.
2. Add all remaining ingredients to oil / flour mixture and bring to a gentle boil.
3. Once mixture boils, turn heat to low and simmer gently until sauce is thickened, about 5 minutes.

Huevos Rancheros Option:

This sauce is delicious and makes outstanding Huevos Rancheros.

Just mix up a batch, heat up an organic corn tortilla and organic refried beans and cook a couple eggs over easy, top the tortilla with beans, eggs, hot enchilada sauce and a couple slices of avocado. Yum!

MICHELE'S MEXICAN BUTTERNUT SQUASH ENCHILADAS

Yields: 8 – 10 Enchiladas

Make **Mexican Butternut Squash** filling recipe on page 224. Make 1 batch of **Outstanding Home-Made Enchilada Sauce** page 246 or use your favorite sauce.

8 – 10 organic corn tortillas.

Assembly Directions:

1. Preheat oven to 350 F.
2. Layer a 13 x 9 casserole dish with parchment paper or, lightly spray with coconut oil.
3. Heat sauce in fry pan or wide-mouth sauce pan until hot and boiling gently.
4. Remove sauce from heat and carefully submerge one corn tortilla for only a few seconds to heat and soften the tortilla, not cook it.
5. Remove the sauce softened tortilla and place on plate.
6. Scoop a few tablespoons of filling onto the center of the tortilla and fold over. Using a spatula, begin making a row of enchiladas in your prepared casserole dish.
7. Once your baking dish is filled with rolled enchiladas, spoon more sauce over each enchilada and bake in 350 F. degree oven for approximately 30 minutes, or until enchiladas are hot.
8. Top with a dollop of organic non-dairy yogurt and a scoop of guacamole, or slices of avocado.

MICHELE'S MARVELOUS MEXICAN CASSEROLE

Yield: Family Size - 12 - 15 servings
Make ½ batch for smaller crowd.
You can also make full recipe, split in two and freeze second half for another time.

Ingredients:

- 2 cups quinoa cooked to package directions
- 1 Tbsp. organic olive oil
- 1 medium/large chopped purple onion
- 2 Tbsp. crushed garlic
- 1 bunch diced green onions
- ½ bunch chopped cilantro - or parsley
- ½ cup organic tomato sauce
- ¾ cup vegetable broth
- 1 can (14 oz.) can black olives, sliced
- 1 can (4 oz.) diced green chilies
- 1 can (14.5) fire roasted tomatoes *(or regular)*
- 1 can (15.25 oz.) organic corn *(or 1 ½ cup frozen)*
- 1 can (15 oz.) organic black beans; kidney beans also work well
- 3 Tbsp. chili powder *(It's fun to experiment here; try 1 teaspoon chipotle & 1 tablespoon Mexican Red & 1/2 teaspoon Ancho Chili)*
- 2 - 3 Tbsp. cumin; Adjust according to taste
- 2 tsp crushed dried oregano
- 2 tsp pink Himalayan salt
- ½ tsp black pepper *(optional)*
- ½ tsp cayenne for heat - optional & to your taste
- 12 pack organic corn tortillas

Enchilada Sauce:

Make a double batch of ***Outstanding Home Made Enchilada Sauce*** recipe page 246 – Or, combine the following to make a tasty, easy enchilada sauce:

- 1 large (1lb 12 oz.) can red chili enchilada sauce
- 1 large (1lb 12 oz.) can green enchilada sauce

Directions:

1. Cook quinoa according to package directions.
2. Open & combine both cans of enchilada sauce and heat in a medium size sauce pan & reserve until it is time to assemble casserole.
3. Sauté purple onion in olive oil or coconut oil until tender
4. Add garlic stir to heat
5. Add each vegetable in order below & mix thoroughly after each addition:
6. Add cilantro (parsley)
7. Add green onion
8. Add roasted, diced tomatoes & mix well
9. Add cooked quinoa
10. Add beans & corn
11. Add seasonings - taste and adjust seasons to your pallet
12. Slice corn tortillas into rectangles

Assembly:

1. 9 X 13 casserole pan; lightly spray with coconut oil.
2. Pour small amount of enchilada sauce into bottom of casserole dish and spread until bottom is covered with thin layer of sauce.
3. Layer half of quinoa mixture on the bottom of the pan.
4. Place single layer of cut tortillas evenly over the filling.
5. Cover tortillas with sauce, making sure all tortillas are covered.
6. Top with remaining 1/2 of quinoa mixture.
7. Top with an additional layer of tortillas.
8. Top tortilla layer with sauce.

Bake at 350 F. for about 30 – 45 minutes or until casserole is hot and cooked through.

SMOKEY BBQ JERK SPICE VEGAN BURGERS

There are tons of veggie patty combinations out there – the imagination goes wild when seeking to create a fun and satisfying meatless burger. The flavors in this recipe are great. Meatless patties do not have the same texture as animal food patties so it takes some getting used to.

Yields: 6 – 8 burger patties

Ingredients:

- 2 – 3 large sweet potatoes; peeled, *cooked & mashed to yield 2 cups*
- ½ cup walnuts; diced & dry roasted; *per directions*
- ½ cup hulled sunflower seeds; chopped and dry roasted; *per directions*
- 1 Tbsp. minced garlic
- ½ onion, diced
- 1 can black beans, rinsed and drained
- ½ tsp salt (*Omit salt if using homemade Jerk Spice recipe*)
- 1 tsp onion powder
- 2 tsp stone ground mustard
- 2 tsp liquid smoke
- ¼ cup gluten-free flour such as tapioca, rice, millet or quinoa
- 2 Tbsp. Jerk Spice seasoning; homemade recipe on page 165, or store bought
- 3 Tbsp. organic ketchup
- Crushed black pepper to taste
- 2 – 3 organic brown-rice cakes, crumpled into small pieces with a few pulses in a food processor or blender – be careful not to turn this into powder, you want a crispy, crunchy texture. Or, use 1 cup GF breadcrumbs.

Directions:

1. Preheat oven to 375 F. Line cookie sheet with parchment paper.
2. Cut 2 – 3 large sweet potatoes in half. Wrap in foil and bake on cookie sheet for 20-30 mins until soft. Peel, mash and set aside.
3. In a small skillet, dry roast the walnuts and hulled sunflower seeds. Be careful not to burn. Watch and remove from heat as soon as nuts begin to yellow on edges. Add to large mixing bowl.
4. Sauté onion & garlic in small amount of vegetable broth until translucent and transfer to mixing bowl with nuts.
5. Mash rinsed, drained black beans with a pastry blender or large fork. You want to keep the beans slightly intact; some mashed, some not so mashed. Add beans to mixing bowl with nuts.
6. Add the 2 cups cooked mashed sweet potato and all remaining ingredients into mixing bowl. Use a large fork and combine thoroughly.
7. Shape mixture into patties and place on parchment lined cookie sheet.
8. Bake at 375 F. for 15 minutes. Remove from oven, carefully turn-over, and cook additional 15 – 20 minutes until slightly crisp around the edges and cooked through.
9. Cool for 5 minutes on cookie rack to help burgers 'set.'
10. Add favorite burger toppings and serve.

➢ **Tip:** *Patties can be served on mashed potatoes with a side of peas or vegetable of choice. Or, lettuce-style wrapped up with tomatoes, pickles, mustard and ketchup. If your body can tolerate eggs, below is a great gluten-free bun recipe you can enjoy. Experiment with what works for you.*

KETO-KING'S GLUTEN-FREE HAMBURGER BUNS

These buns are AMAZING!!! They are the best GF buns we've tried so far. I've added the link here for you to watch the recipe creator "Keto King" in action as he makes these wonderful buns. These buns are gluten-free but contain eggs, so they are not acceptable during the EDD. These buns are a low-carb, grain-free Paleo dieter's delight!

Keto King's YouTube Video: https://www.youtube.com/watch?v=KdhXQ2c5fCk

Yields: 4 – 5 buns; depending on how large you fashion them

Ingredients:

- ¼ cup coconut flour
- ¼ cup almond flour; *not almond meal*
- ¼ flax seed meal; *ground into powder using a coffee grinder*
- 4 eggs; separate 3 eggs; use whites of 3, and 1 whole egg
- Dash sea salt
- 1 tsp organic apple cider vinegar
- 3 Tbsp. finely ground psyllium husk powder; *use coffee grinder*
- 1 tsp baking powder
- 1 tsp onion powder
- 1 cup water
- Either sesame seeds or dry onion flakes to top buns

Directions:

1. Add all dry ingredients to a mixing bowl and thoroughly whisk to blend.
2. Separate three eggs, using only whites, plus one whole egg; whisk to blend.
3. Add water and apple cider vinegar to eggs and whisk to blend.
4. Add liquid to dry ingredients, whisk to blend thoroughly, but be careful not to over mix here as it adds air pockets in the buns.
5. Dough is thick, scoop bun portions onto a parchment paper lined baking sheet. Carefully shape into round buns using the back of a large spoon, or spatula, or your fingers. The shape you put them into the oven is the shape they will stay. They will puff up nicely when baked.

6. Top with either sesame seeds or dry onion flakes for an authentic looking and tasting burger bun. Press seeds or flakes gently to dough to stick while baking.
7. Bake at 350 F. for 50 minutes. Buns will spring gently to the touch when cooked.
8. Place on rack to cool thoroughly before slicing. Buns have a nice texture, and can be sliced and toasted. Fill with your favorite meatless burger or sandwich fixings and enjoy!

➤ **Tip:** This recipe can be adapted for a variety of applications. Fill them with the 'Mock-Tuna' Chickpea filling, or for a sweet touch, try the recipe below.

<u>Cinnamon Walnut Breakfast Scones</u>:

Follow above directions omitting the onion powder, seeds & onion flakes.

Add to dry ingredients:

- 1 tsp cinnamon
- ½ tsp nutmeg
- ½ tsp allspice
- ¼ tsp cloves
- ¼ cup finely chopped walnuts
- ¼ cup raisins

Add to wet ingredients:

- 1 Tbsp. pure maple syrup, or raw honey
- 1 tsp pure vanilla extract

Follow the above instructions but shape the dough into oblong scone shapes rather than round buns. Sprinkle with cinnamon and bake at 350 F. for 50 minutes. Serve warm if desired. Or, once fully cooled, scones can be sliced, toasted and topped with favorite low-sugar jam or jelly.

ON THE SWEET SIDE

GLUTEN FREE APPLE CINNAMON COFFEE CAKE

Yields: One 8-inch coffee cake; approximately 8 servings

Ingredients:

- 2 large organic apples peeled, cored & diced. If apples are small, use 3.
- 5 Tbsp. melted coconut oil & separated in half
- 3 Tbsp. coconut sugar
- 2 Tbsp. maple syrup
- 3 large eggs; room temperature
- ½ cup coconut or almond non-dairy milk
- 4 tsp cinnamon; 2 tsp in apple topping, 2 tsp in coffee cake batter
- 1 Tbsp. pure vanilla
- 2 cups almond flour – *not* almond meal
- ½ cup gluten free flour; i.e. *Pamela's Artisan*, or *Bob's Red Mill*
- ½ tsp sea salt
- ½ tsp nutmeg
- ¼ tsp allspice
- dash cloves
- 2 tsp baking powder
- 1 tsp baking soda

Directions:

1. Preheat oven to 350 F. Line the bottom of an 8-inch cake pan with parchment paper. Or, use an 8-inch spring form pan; lightly sprayed with coconut spray.

2. Melt coconut oil and separate in half; you will be using half in the apple topping, and half in the coffee cake batter.

3. Peel, core and *dice* the two large apples; or 3 small. Using *half* the coconut oil (2 ½ Tbsp.) add apples, 2 tsp cinnamon, 2 Tbsp. maple syrup and 2 Tbsp. of water into a small sauce pan and sauté apples until soft being careful not to burn. Add a *tiny* bit more water if necessary. You do not want this watery, but rather a nice cinnamon glaze that cooks the apples. It is helpful to cook this mixture in a double-boiler if you have one.

4. Once apples are *soft* and cooked *completely*, mash apples a bit with a large fork, or pastry blender until apples pieces resemble chunky applesauce. Separate in half, one half for topping, and one half to be added to the cake batter wet ingredients.

5. **Apple Topping**: Reserve *half* the apple mixture for apple cake topping.

6. **Wet Batter Ingredients**: Mix together the second half of the mashed apples with all the wet ingredients; three eggs, 2 ½ Tbsps. melted coconut oil, 1/2 cup non-dairy milk, and 1 Tbsps. vanilla. Whisk to combine thoroughly.

7. **Dry Batter Ingredients:** In a separate bowl, add all dry ingredients: 2 cups almond flour, ½ cup gluten-free flour, 3 Tbsp. coconut sugar, ½ tsp salt, 2 tsp cinnamon, ½ tsp nutmeg, ¼ tsp allspice, dash cloves, 1 tsp baking powder and ½ tsp baking soda. Whisk until blended.

8. Combine wet ingredients with dry and mix thoroughly to blend. Pour cake batter into prepared pan. Then, carefully spread the cooked apple cinnamon topping over the coffee cake batter. Bake at 350 F. for approximately 30 – 40 minutes. Coffee cake is done when toothpick comes out clean.

9. Let cake cool about 15 – 20 minutes on rack. Serve warm or cooled.

For best results refrigerate left-over coffee cake. It keeps real well in the fridge for 3 – 4 days.

Option: APPLE-CINNAMON BREAD PUDDING

Use all the same ingredients and follow directions on previous page – *except* you are NOT going to *separate* the cooked apple chunks. *And*, you are NOT going to mash the apples. Leave the cooked apples in chunks and add all the cooked apples to the wet ingredients.

Mix all the dry ingredients together and whisk to blend. Then add the apple, egg wet ingredient mixture to the dry ingredients and combine thoroughly for a thick, apple-chunky batter.

Here are two suggestions for cooking the apple-cinnamon bread pudding:

1. Casserole Pudding Instructions: Pour batter in a greased 8-inch casserole dish, uncovered for about 30 – 40 minutes. Pudding is cooked when toothpick comes out clean.

2. Individual Ramekins: Lightly spray ramekins with coconut oil spray and fill each to ¾ capacity. Bake 15 minutes. Pudding is cooked when toothpick comes out clean.

Top Apple-Cinnamon Bread Pudding with **Coconut Whip Cream** recipe page 261.

RAW CHOCOLATE PEANUTBUTTER CREAM PIE

Another crowd-dazzling GLUTEN FREE, raw, dairy free, egg free treat sure to please any crowd!

Yields: 8-10 servings, very rich, make serving sizes small

Ingredients:

- 1 ½ cups raw – soaked – cashews. Cover cashews with boiling water and soak for at least 15 minutes; then drain.
- 1 cup organic peanut butter; chunky or smooth – doesn't matter
- ½ cup water
- ¾ cup organic cocoa powder
- 1 Tbsp. pure vanilla extract
- ¾ cup pure maple syrup or ½ cu raw honey
- ¼ cup coconut oil
- ¼ tsp fine sea salt

Directions:

1. Prepare **Raw Nut & Date Pie Crust** page 265 . *Option;* use peanuts for nuts.
2. In heavy-duty blender or food processor combine drained cashews, ½ cup water, vanilla, maple syrup & salt until completely smooth, no chunks. Stop a couple times, use a spatula and scrape down sides continuing until smooth.
3. Add peanut butter and coconut oil, and blend to incorporate.
4. Add chocolate and blend. This mixture will be very thick and sticky; stop often and scrape sides. The longer you blend this mixture the lighter it becomes.
5. Taste and adjust sweetness.
6. Pour into prepared crust and freeze at least one hour before serving.

Keep in the freezer. Chocolate pie slices well frozen.

GLUTEN FREE CINNAMON CRUMBLE BANANA MUFFINS

Yields: 12 muffins

Ingredients:

- 3 ripe bananas, mashed
- ¼ cup maple syrup
- 1 tsp vanilla
- 3 eggs, whisked together
- ½ cup almond butter
- ¾ cup coconut flour
- 1 tsp baking soda
- 1 tsp baking powder
- 1 tsp cinnamon
- ½ teaspoon nutmeg
- ¼ allspice
- ½ teaspoon salt

Cinnamon Crumble Topping

- ¼ cup coconut oil; softened with fork, do not melt.
- 2 Tbsp. coconut sugar
- 2 Tbsp. almond meal, or flour
- 1 tsp cinnamon
- ½ tsp allspice
- ½ cup pecans or walnuts, crushed

Mix ingredients together until crumbled; set aside.

Directions:

1. Preheat oven to 350 F. & line 12-piece muffin pan with cupcake papers.
2. Mix together cinnamon topping ingredients until nice and crumbled. I find a small food processor works great to get a nice, crumbled consistency. Just pulse until crumbly – over mixing will produce paste so be careful.
3. In a large bowl, mix together bananas, maple, vanilla extract, eggs, and almond butter. Whisk, or beat, together until all ingredients are well blended.

4. Combine dry ingredients; coconut flour, baking powder, baking soda, cinnamon & spices, salt and mix well.

5. Add dry ingredients to wet and mix until nice and lumpy gooey - then drop evenly into 12-piece muffin tin. This batter will be very thick and should fill a 12-piece muffin pan perfectly.

6. Top each muffin with cinnamon topping mixture & bake approx. 15 - 18 minutes. A toothpick inserted in the middle should come out free of dough crumbs when done.

MOM'S FAVORITE PUMPKIN PIE

Recently, my Mom was with us in the mountains for a beautiful, restful vacation - and she bit into our delicious pumpkin pie and said *"Wow! This is the best pumpkin pie I have had this season! Where did you get the recipe?"*

This recipe is our own creation - enjoy!

Yields: 1 pie - 8 slices

Pie Filling Ingredients:

- One 15-ounce can unsweetened pure organic pumpkin
- One 11.25 ounce can <u>sweetened condensed coconut milk</u> - This is the **secret ingredient** right here! Available at Sprouts & Wholefoods. Or online. No additional sugar is necessary for this recipe. This makes for a creamy, light texture.
- 3 eggs lightly beaten
- 1 ½ tsp cinnamon
- ½ tsp sea salt
- ½ tsp ground ginger
- ½ tsp allspice
- ¼ tsp ground nutmeg
- ¼ tsp cloves

Perfect Flaky Pie Crust:

- 1 ½ cups organic palm shortening
- 3 cups all-purpose organic unbleached white flour. Or, *Pamela's Gluten-Free Artisan* white flour
- 1 whole egg; beaten
- 5 Tbsp. cold water
- 1 Tbsp. plain white vinegar
- 1 tsp sea salt

This recipe makes two pie crusts for regular size 10-inch pies. Or, separate dough into three equal pieces for a thinner crust and wrap and freeze remaining dough for your next pie!

Pie Directions:
1. Mix all ingredients together in a medium mixing bowl.
2. Pour mixture into a prepared pie crust.
3. Bake at 400 F for initial 15 minutes, turn oven down to 350 F. and cook additional 1 to 1 ¼ hours. Pie is done when toothpick inserted into center comes out clean.

Crust Directions:

1. In food processor mix flour, shortening and salt together in pulsing bursts until flour mixture resembles small peas, or course meal.
2. Mix wet ingredients together, and add liquid through top of processor bowl a little at a time until incorporated into a ball.
3. Separate ball into 2 – or 3 portions, depending on how thick you want the dough. Press ball slightly to flatten, wrap in saran and either freeze until ready to use, or freeze 15 – 20 minutes in order to chill before rolling out into a crust.

Top pie with this delicious non-dairy whip cream.

Coconut Whip Cream

- 1 can cold full-fat coconut cream. Refrigerate for at least 24-hours.
- 1 tsp vanilla
- 1 tsp cinnamon
- 2 Tbsp. Maple syrup

Open can and carefully scoop off thick cream. Using mixer, whip cream, vanilla, cinnamon and syrup until thick and creamy.

RAW DOUBLE-LAYER CHOCOLATE FUDGE

Dazzle your non-vegan friends with this delicious treat and they will never doubt your ability to create tasty and healthy treats!

Yields: 16 - 20 small squares

Ingredients:

FOR THE FUDGE LAYER:

- 1 cup raw walnut pieces
- ½ cup hulled hemp seeds
- 1 ½ cups pitted Medjool dates
- ½ cup raw cacao powder
- 1 ½ tsp pure vanilla extract
- ¼ teaspoon pink Himalayan salt or fine grain sea salt
- Heaping 2 Tbsp. raw cacao nibs; or organic chocolate chips
- Heaping ¼ cup raw walnut pieces

FOR THE HOMEMADE CHOCOLATE TOPPING:

- ½ cup coconut oil
- ½ cup raw cacao powder or organic cocoa powder
- ¼ cup pure maple syrup
- small pinch fine grain sea salt
- ¼ tsp pure vanilla extract

Directions:

1. For the fudge bottom layer: Line an 8-inch square pan with parchment paper, one piece going each way to make it easy to lift fudge out later on.
2. In a food processor, process the walnuts into a fine crumb - remove and set aside for step 5.
3. Add the hemp seeds and the pitted dates and process until finely chopped and sticky. Mixture will be very thick and gooey in texture.
4. Add the cacao powder, vanilla, and pink salt and process until thoroughly combined.
5. Stir or pulse in the cacao nibs and chopped walnuts until just combined.

6. Evenly press the mixture into prepared square pan. Use a spatula, or the back of a large mixing spoon to flatten mixture and spread evenly on the bottom of the pan making a smooth layer. Place in the freezer for about 10 minutes.

7. For the chocolate topping: Melt the coconut oil over low heat in a medium pan. Remove from heat and whisk in the cacao powder, syrup, salt, and vanilla until combined and smooth.

8. Remove the fudge from the freezer and pour chocolate topping over base. Spread evenly. Carefully transfer the pan to the freezer on a flat, even surface. Chill for 20 + minutes or until the topping is firm enough to slice.

9. After fudge is frozen cut into servings sizes and keep remaining pieces frozen in a zip-lock baggie.

10. To slice, lift frozen fudge out of the pan using the parchment paper handles and set on flat surface. Run hot water over a knife for a minute or so, wipe quickly with towel, and carefully slide the knife into the fudge to slice. Warming up the knife helps it slice more evenly without much cracking.

Store leftover in the freezer for a chocolate treat anytime!

RAW STRAWBERRY CREAM PIE

Gluten Free, dairy free, egg free
Yields: 6 - 8 servings

Ingredients:

- 2 ½ cups raw – soaked – cashews. Cover cashews with boiling water and soak for at least 15 minutes; then drain.
- 1 Tbsp. pure vanilla extract
- ½ cup pure maple syrup or ½ cup raw honey
- ¼ cup melted coconut oil
- ½ cup fresh lemon juice
- 1 – 2 tsp lemon zest *(grate lemon peel on fine mesh side of grater for zest)*
- ¼ cup water
- Dash fine sea salt
- Fresh organic berries of choice – or frozen berries

STRAWBERRY TOPPING: Wash, de-stem and chop about 2 cups of fresh organic strawberries. Blend strawberries with a little maple syrup or raw honey for sauce. If using a medley of frozen berries just set them out for a little while to defrost and mottle slightly (*mush them up*) to create a yummy berry sauce topping.

Directions:

1. Combine cashews and ¼ cup water in a heavy-duty blender or food processor. Blend until cashews are smooth, no chunks.
2. Add remaining ingredients and continue to process for 6 – 7 minutes, stopping occasionally to scrape sides. The longer you blend this mixture the lighter it becomes.
3. Taste and adjust sweetness, add a little more sweet or lemon to suit your taste.
4. Pour into prepared **Raw Nut & Date Pie Crust** page 265. Freeze prepared pie for at least one hour before serving.
5. After pie is frozen slice and top with berries and serve. Keep frozen, pie cuts well frozen. It's a delightful treat – almost takes the place of ice cream. *Almost.*

Banana Cream Pie *Option*: Add one banana to above ingredients and process as above. Top with **Coconut Whip Cream** page 261.

Chocolate Cream Pie *Option*: Omit lemon. Add cashews and all liquid to food processor and mix until cashews are creamy. Then, add ¾ cup unsweetened, organic cocoa powder and process until creamy and incorporated. Mixture will be sticky. You should not see any cashew bits in mixture. Additional water and sweetener are needed when using chocolate, taste and add as needed. Top with **Coconut Whip Cream** page 261.

RAW NUT & DATE PIE CRUST *(gluten-free)*

This DELICIOUS gluten-free raw pie crust works well with any pie that calls for a graham cracker crust.

- About ¾ cup pitted dates
- ½ cup chopped nuts; your choice; almonds, pecans or walnuts
- dash salt
- 1 tsp pure vanilla extract
- Up to 1 Tbsp. water, if needed

Line a round 8-inch spring form pan with parchment paper, and set aside.

If you do not have a spring form pan, lightly grease an 8-inch pie dish with coconut oil.

Combine all crust ingredients except water in a high-quality food processor *(not blender)* until fine crumbles form. If mixture is too dry, add the water. Press the crust mixture into the prepared pan. If mixture is thick and difficult to spread, dampen your fingertips and press gently to spread evenly over the bottom of pie dish. Cover and freeze until ready to use.

Body Speak!

Chapter 20
RELIABLE HEALTH RESOURCES

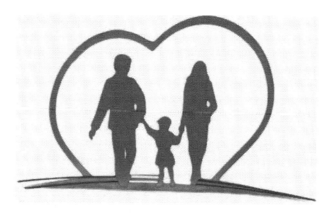

In my research for answers and the truth about health and nutrition, I searched for doctors and health professionals with LONG histories of actually healing their patients and clients.

Here you will find experts in the field of nutrition, natural healing protocols and laboratories that produce pure, high-potency and reliable 'nutraceuticals' that heal and detoxify the body.

Check out my Health Coach Website – I will keep updating this list and putting links to the latest information and science backed health articles. I'm available for personal health coaching sessions. Together we will work on successfully achieving your health goals www.michelemrizzo.com.

Coach Michele's Personal Programs

Michele's health programs include group coaching classes, health retreats, half-day health seminars and six-week workshops. Michele teaches periodic live online courses and cooking classes – *Check it out at: www.michelemrizzo.com.*

Michele offers private six-month coaching programs where she works with clients to help them create specific goals and achieve optimum health and well-being.

As an Integrative Health Coach Michele weaves all aspects of life into her coaching practice including; nutrition, relationships, career, self-help and spirituality. Life is more than the food on your plate!

Michele empowers her clients and students to create happy, healthy lives in a way that is flexible, fun and sustainable. She works with people to help them discover the food and lifestyle choices that will best support them and their life and health goals.

Michele offer's complementary Health History Consultations. Spend a pleasant 60 minutes with Michele discussing your health goals: *http://michelemrizzo.com/pages/health-coaching*

- A FEW CLIENT TESTIMONIALS -

"Michele met me right where I am and never shamed me for my perspectives and my struggles. Michele didn't try to convince me about what was right or wrong or good or bad in my various approaches, she very much respected my personal journey of success and failure. Not only do I feel understood and supported but I am a having success in reaching my health goals!" – Kristin, WI

"The changes are huge! I can't stop smiling. I needed someone who saw the jewel inside me even though I was tired and had started to give up. Michele, thank you for helping me, thank you for encouraging me, and thank you for walking through this journey with me." – Marie, TX

"Michele answered my many questions, helping me focus on new menus, nutritional supplements and new goals. As we talked and I used the tools Michele offered, I found myself getting better each day. I am enjoying wearing the clothes that have been in my closet for a couple of years, because of the 21 pounds I've lost in less than six weeks!" – Joyce, CA

MICHELE IS AVAILABLE FOR SPEAKING TEACHING & COOKING CLASSES

Michele will tailor health classes, half or full-day seminars and / or cooking classes to suit the needs of your business, organization, or a gathering of your favorite family & friends. Contact Michele today for more information: Michele@michclemrizzo.com.

BECOME A PROFESSIONAL HEALTH COACH!

BODY SPEAK! Was inspired by Michele's experience attending the Institute of Integrative Nutrition ® (IIN), where she received her training in holistic wellness and health coaching. IIN offers a truly comprehensive Health Coach Training Program that invites students to deeply explore the things that are most nourishing to them.

Beyond personal health, IIN offers training in health coaching, as well as business and marketing. Students who choose to pursue this field professionally complete the program equipped with communication skills and branding knowledge they need to create a fulfilling career encouraging and supporting others in reaching their own health goals.

Feel free to contact Michele to hear more about her personal experience at IIN. You can copy & paste the following personalized Ambassador link into your browser for a brochure of how you can become a professional Health Coach:

```
<a target="newwin" href="http://geti.in/2bD1Vpw"> <img style="width:250px;"
src="https://www.shareiin.com/sites/default/files/DES_749_New_Ambassador_Instagram_C_0.jpg?id=00138
000018FFX7AAO"/> </a>
```

Or, call (844) 315-8546 & be sure to mention Michele M. Rizzo referred you!

CANCER RESOURCES

"THE THUTH ABOUT" – TTAC Series – Ty Bollinger

Ty Bollinger, best-selling author, medical researcher, talk radio host and health freedom advocate has created a series of ground-breaking, revolutionizing and educational exposes' on the truth about cancer, detox and vaccines.

After losing several family members to cancer (including his mother and father), Ty refused to accept the notion that chemotherapy, radiation, and surgery were the most effective treatments available for cancer patients. He began a quest to learn all he possibly could about alternative cancer treatments and the medical industry.

Ty's quest for the truth has evolved into the most informative, cutting edge, science based information on today's most critical health issues.

If you or a love one is battling cancer – Ty Bollinger's **Truth About Cancer – A Global Quest** – is a MUST! This docuseries will educate you, give you hope and launch you into finding the best approach for overcoming cancer by healing your body and strengthening your immune system:

https://www.cancertutor.com/global-cancer-documentary/

The TRUTH about CANCER – official YouTube channel. Good stuff!
https://www.youtube.com/user/thetruthaboutcancer

The TRUTH about CANCER – Facebook Page:
https://www.facebook.com/thetruthaboutcancer/videos/899347643491879/

"Cancer the Forbidden Cures" - Excellent & Informative Documentary

This documentary opened my eyes to the truth about the history of cancer cures that have been purposely hidden from the public for decades. The American Medical Associate (AMA), the pharmaceutical industry, and the cancer industry – do not want people to understand there are natural, proven cures for cancer. Watch this documentary and learn the truth for yourself:

https://www.youtube.com/watch?v=NAMYAoiCSsI&t=62s

In this documentary they talk about how Essiac tea helped cure cancer in the early 1900's. Here is a link to an informative article about Essiac tea, and how to make it: https://thetruthaboutcancer.com/essiac-tea-cancer-fighting/

Baking Soda Found to Cure Fungal Related Cancer:

Dr. Jan told Mike to drink a baking soda mixture along with cumin oil and organic black strap molasses. We had no idea why, but we did it. Later on, we discovered why. Professor Tullia Simoncini, Italian Oncologist, discovered baking soda melts malignant tumors. Prof Simoncini thought he would be hailed as a breakthrough genius for finding a cure for cancer, but instead he was professionally ostracized, criticized, attacked and his medical license was threatened if he continued:

Prof Simoncini's website: *http://www.curenaturalicancro.com/en/*

YouTube Interview: *https://www.youtube.com/watch?v=5XdgNYiOcp8*

DETOX & Healing Chronic Illness

TTAC – The Truth about Detox: This is an excellent and informative series on how to undergo a seven-day full body detox. This program offers high-quality nutraceutical products you can purchase to intensify a thorough detox protocol: *https://thetruthaboutdetox.com/1/insider-access/*

Dr. Robert Morse's Herbal Health Club. Dr. Morse has been reversing chronic disease and healing cancer for forty years. His video series are full of information and instructions on how to detox and heal the body from every disease and disorder.

> **Video**: - *The Simplicity of Cancer*:
> *https://www.drmorsesherbalhealthclub.com/blogs/media/60014405-the-simplicity-of-cancer*
>
> **Book:** *The Detox Miracle Sourcebook: Raw Foods and Herbs for*

Body Speak!

> ### *Complete Cellular Regeneration:*
>
> *https://www.amazon.com/Detox-Miracle-Sourcebook-Complete-Regeneration/dp/1935826190/ref=sr_1_1?ie=UTF8&qid=1504389633&sr=8-1&keywords=robert+Morse*

EDUCATIONAL HEALTH & NUTRITION

Dr. Robert Scott Bell – THE POWER TO HEAL IS YOURS!
http://www.robertscottbell.com/

Dr. Joseph Mercola is a trustworthy voice in functional medicine, nutrition and natural healing. Here is a link to his vast video library:
http://articles.mercola.com/videos.aspx

Dr. John McDougall – physician, author, nutrition expert; healing thousands of people for decades. https://www.drmcdougall.com/about/dr-john-mcdougall/

Dr. Joel Fuhrman – physician, author, wholefood, plant based nutrition expert. Dr. Fuhrman's newest book is entitled; "Fast Food Genocide,"
https://www.drfuhrman.com/?gclid=Cj0KEQjwranNBRDh3uGN5ojp9o8BEiQASu908KuauM21oX-HkjFNNfyTzWMevdMYdgP9qA3NbTJvmYUaAihy8P8HAQ

RELIABLE - LABS FOR NUTRACEUTICALS & SUPPLEMENTS

Mike Adams – the Health Ranger – is a food forensic scientist and health advocate. His website is full of cutting edge information on true scientific advances, as well as exposing the false information out there regarding health politics and misinformation. http://www.naturalnews.com/About.html

Mike Adams is a reliable source for pure, high-grade supplements and nutraceuticals. Health Ranger products: https://www.healthrangerstore.com/

Dr. Edward F. Group – Founder – The Global Healing Center; Dr. Group is a nutritional health expert and creator of high-potency, pure nutraceuticals & supplements. https://www.globalhealingcenter.com/about/dr-group

RECIPE INDEX

EDD BREAKFAST SELECTIONS

Smoothie Recipes:

Berry Blend Delight	181
Frothy Banana Strawberry Fruit Smoothie	181
Health Blast Juice!	184
Heavenly Green Smoothie	183
Powerhouse Punch Green Smoothie	182

Breakfast Entrée Selections:

Ginger Millet Skillet	189
Overnight Oatmeal	185
Pumpkin Pie Rice Pudding	188
RAW Apple Compote	186
Rice Cream Dream	187
Sweet Potato Country Hash	190
UPMA – Traditional Indian Breakfast	191

EDD LUNCH ENTRÉE SELECTIONS

EDD Oil - Free Salad Dressings:

Fat-free Cilantro Zucchini	192
Balsamic Vinaigrette	194
Creamy Vinaigrette	193
Sweet Tangy Thai	193
Vegan Ranch	194

Hummus & Salsa:

Delicious Oil-Free Hummus!	204
Mango Salsa	202
Roasted Tomatillo Salsa Verde	199

EDD Salad Entrée Selections

Crunchy Broccoli Salad	196
Mediterranean Style Quinoa Salad	198
Mexican Veggie & Bean Salad	197
Mock Tuna Chickpea Salad Wraps	195
RAW Master Vegetable Salad	135
Vegan Taco Salad	200

EDD Savory Soup Entrée Selections

Cream of Asparagus Soup	206
Creamy Cheesy Broccoli Soup	207
Old Fashion Split Pea Potato Soup	209
Quick-Soak Beans Method	162
Savory Lentil Soup	228
Simple Black Bean Soup	212
Spicy Bean & Sweet Potato Soup	210
Sweet Spicy Thai Noodle Soup	208
Vegetable Minestrone Soup	205

EDD MAIN MEAL ENTRÉE & SIDE SELECTIONS

Sides to Top with Vegetable Stir Fries & Stews:

Cauliflower Fried Rice	213
Herb & Veggie Brown Rice with Mushrooms & Capers	216
Quinoa Pilaf	215
Tasty Mashed Potatoes	214
Vegan Cashew Cheese	231

Main Entrée's:

Easy Delicious Simple Quinoa Chili	226
Delicious Gluten-Free Vegan Pizza	230

Gluten-Free Pizza Crust   230

Indian-Spiced Veggie Medley   229

Italian Pizza / Marinara Sauce   230

Kung Pao Cauliflower Stir-Fry   234

Lentil Artichoke Stew   222

Louisiana-Style Red Beans & Rice   220

Mexican Butternut Squash   224

Mexican Lentil Chili   217

Mushroom Lentil Bourguignon   223

Outstanding Enchilada Sauce   246

Potato Cauliflower Curry   218

Thai Veggie Sauté   219

AFTER EDD DELICIOUS HEALTHY RECIPES

A Few 'Go-to' Favorites

These recipes are gluten-free (GF), some contain eggs, corn & nuts.

Breakfast Selections:

GF Apple Upside-down Coffee Cake	254
GF Apple Cinnamon Bread Pudding	256
GF Cinnamon Nut Bread	240
GF Cinnamon-Crumble Banana Muffins	258
GF Oat Pancakes	242
GF Breakfast Scones	253
Huevos Rancheros – *Option*	246

Lunch & Dinner Selections:

Italian Mac N'Cheese	244
Jerk Spice Seasoning	165
Keto-Hamburger Buns	252
Michele's Mexican Butternut Enchiladas	247
Michele's Marvelous Mexican Casserole	248
Outstanding Homemade Enchilada Sauce	246
Potluck Salad	245
Smokey BBQ Jerk Spice Vegan Hamburger Patties	250
Vegan Mac N'Cheese	243

On The Sweet Side:

Coconut Non-Dairy Whip Cream	261
Mom's Favorite Pumpkin Pie	260
RAW Double-Layer Chocolate Fudge	262
RAW Banana Cream Pie	265
RAW Chocolate Cream Pie	265
RAW Chocolate Peanut Butter Cream Pie	257
RAW Nut & Date Pie Crust	265
RAW Strawberry Cream Pie	264